'Written in a comprehensive yet simple and accessible manner, *Hypnotherapy with Regrets and Associated Emotions: Ideas for Practice* is a highly applicable, generalisable and useful text. The content is excellent and very thorough and well written. It contains a useful chapter explaining how to use the diverse ideas for working with both children and adults, and a very large range of type or regrets covering all areas. The scripts themselves are thorough and well written and provoke other ideas in the reader. There is a wide and varied theme for the scripts providing something suitable for every client and their style/ interests. Most significantly, I like the encouragement for practitioners to apply some of the book to themselves through self-reflection. I certainly intend to use and suggest that any hypnotherapists that I train purchase this unique book.'

**Caroline Dyson**, *Founder and Director of Hypnotherapy in Schools Programme (HISP) and Managing Minds (MM), hypnotherapist, psychotherapist and trainer*

# Hypnotherapy with Regrets and Associated Emotions

This book helps hypnotherapists to focus on the subject of regrets and associated emotions when working with clients.

Promoting the concept of "the road of regrets", this book presents a five-stage process for the hypnotherapist to work through with clients (adults and children aged 5+). The process involves identifying and acknowledging regrets; working through the regrets and associated emotions; taking any necessary action before releasing the regrets and emotions; and finally moving on to plan for the future. The book contains over 60 customisable scripts, guidance notes and appendices to promote ideas for practice. The scripts offer a variety of methodology to choose from: regression (including past lives); metaphors (Ericksonian); benefits approach; Gestalt therapy and solution-focused. The appendices include practical resources such as questions and questionnaires, checklists, summaries, forms, and worksheets for exercises which the hypnotherapist can utilise in sessions (individual or group).

This practical volume will be of use to student hypnotherapists, trainers and training schools, supervisors, newly qualified and experienced hypnotherapists. Although the main focus of the book is regrets and associated emotions, the book can be used for an abundance of other concerns e.g. lack of confidence or self-esteem; fears; anxiety and panic attacks.

**Jacki Pritchard** works as a clinical hypnotherapist, independent social worker and trainer in social care. She offers hypnotherapy services to adults and children (age 5+) in two practice locations, schools and colleges.

# Hypnotherapy with Regrets and Associated Emotions

Ideas for Practice

Jacki Pritchard

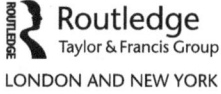

Routledge
Taylor & Francis Group

LONDON AND NEW YORK

Designed cover image: © Getty Images

First published 2025
by Routledge
4 Park Square, Milton Park, Abingdon, Oxon OX14 4RN

and by Routledge
605 Third Avenue, New York, NY 10158

*Routledge is an imprint of the Taylor & Francis Group, an informa business*

© 2025 Jacki Pritchard

*British Library Cataloguing-in-Publication Data*
A catalogue record for this book is available from the British Library

ISBN: 9781032742397 (hbk)
ISBN: 9781032735900 (pbk)
ISBN: 9781003468325 (ebk)

DOI: 10.4324/9781003468325

Typeset in Times New Roman
by Deanta Global Publishing Services, Chennai, India

This book is dedicated to my grand-daughter
Maeve Rose
May your regrets be few through your lifetime

# Contents

# Part I

# Working with regrets

# Chapter 1

# Introduction

## Why we should work with regrets

I am sure most people have heard the saying "Life is too short to have regrets"; and I would totally agree with that statement. Everyone should try to get on and enjoy their life fully – get the most out of it while they can. However, when people say you should not dwell on the past I would not totally agree with this. I am a great reflector and I think it can be enlightening to look back at the past to gain some understanding about what has happened and perhaps analyse behaviours, that is, try to understand why a person did what they did or said what they said. I would agree it is unhealthy to live in the past, but reminiscence does have a place at certain times in one's life. Similarly, thinking about regrets, acknowledging and working through them are a necessity in order to move forward.

These views and comments stem from my experiences working both as a social worker and a clinical hypnotherapist for many years. As a social worker specialising in the abuse of both adults and children, I have always adopted the psychodynamic approach. I believe it is necessary to find the root cause of a problem and address it in order to move on. When I trained to be a hypnotherapist, I was taught many different methods and techniques; and to this day I will always utilise the method which is best for my client. It is very trendy nowadays to advocate being in the present. Hence why cognitive behavioural therapy (CBT) and solution-focused therapy (SFT) have become so popular amongst all types of therapists. Both approaches focus very much on the here and now. In my own practice I do use either approach when it is appropriate for the client. I feel strongly it is important to be person-centred and not restrict oneself in methods utilised. When working with regrets it is important to look at the past and this is one of the reasons I wanted to write this book. I do not think it is helpful to ignore regrets or sweep them under the carpet. Some fundamental questions regarding regrets are – do we:

- Acknowledge them?
- Dismiss them too easily?
- Work with them enough or thoroughly enough?
- Spend sufficient time working through them?

DOI: 10.4324/9781003468325-2

## Reasons for writing the book

In my work as a social worker and hypnotherapist, I frequently have clients (both adults and children) talking about what they regret doing or not doing. This usually comes out during the course of a conversation; either at assessment stage or during a subsequent home visit or therapy session. This has led me to believe, as I have stated above, that it is important to work on regrets – not dismiss them by saying clichés like the one I stated at the beginning of this introduction: "Life is too short to have regrets". When I was writing my last book which was concerned with looking at different types of losses[1], I kept thinking about regrets because there can often be a close link between losses and regrets. When a loss is experienced there can be a feeling of regret, for example, not having done something or told someone how you feel; or a person can question whether they could have done or said anything differently. Although there may be a link between losses and regrets, the two subjects need to be looked at in their own individual right. I do feel that sometimes professionals and workers do not give enough attention or spend sufficient time working on regrets. I believe that the subject of working on regrets needs more attention, to be given some prominence and consequently deserved a book in its own right. So one of the main purposes in putting this book together is to encourage the hypnotherapist to think about their own practice in relation to regrets and before proceeding to read the book ask themselves the following questions:

- When do I think about regrets?
- When did I last think about regrets?
- When did I last consider the emotions associated with regrets?
- Do I give regrets enough attention in the work I do?
- Do I acknowledge regrets when working with clients?
- Do I dismiss regrets too easily?
- Do I work with regrets enough or thoroughly enough?
- Do I spend sufficient time working through regrets with clients?
- What do I need to do to improve my practice in working with regrets?

## Regrets and emotions

In order to work through regrets, it is necessary to focus on the emotions associated with them. In their day-to-day practice the hypnotherapist will be working to look at the links between a client's thoughts, feelings and behaviours. An essential bit of the work is to look at these links, i.e. stop the thoughts, release the negative feelings and change behaviours. The emotions and feelings associated with regrets can have both short-term and long-term effects on a person's life and result in particular issues/problems, which the hypnotherapist is probably dealing with every day in their working life e.g. lack of confidence; low self-esteem; fears; phobias; anxiety and panic attacks. This is discussed more fully in Chapter 4, but it is important to say in this introduction that many of the scripts and visualisations included in the book focus on working with emotions and feelings; and therefore, can be used for other issues/problems presented to the hypnotherapist, not just when working on regrets.

## Objectives of the book

The main objectives of the book are to:

*   Stimulate thinking about the subject of regrets and for the hypnotherapist to question whether they address the subject enough in their own practice
*   Encourage hypnotherapists to be more pro-active in working with regrets i.e. not just when the subject arises with a client who is already having hypnotherapy sessions
*   Consider the different types of regrets a person may experience through their lifetime i.e. from childhood through to the older years (and ultimately death)
*   Focus on emotions associated with regrets by considering the link between thoughts, feelings and behaviours
*   Offer a structured process to work with regrets and the associated emotions
*   Present and discuss ideas for practice when working with regrets and emotions
*   Develop skills in working with regrets and emotions
*   Have a resource of scripts and visualisations (for both adults and children) which have been tried and tested when working with regrets; and which can be used to work with other issues/problems, which the hypnotherapist is presented with in their day-to-day practice
*   Provide questions, questionnaires, checklists, summaries, forms, exercises and worksheets which the hypnotherapist can utilise when working with a client in sessions.

## Who will find the book useful?

The book has been written primarily for:

### *Student hypnotherapists*

Students need to practise and build their confidence as they develop their knowledge and skills. It can be very scary when you start to put the theory into practice, because you never know what the client's subconscious mind is going to bring forward. It can be helpful for a student to read scripts to get an understanding of how they can be written in different ways, but also how they can be used to practise. Preparation and practise is an essential part of the learning process in order to become an effective and skilled hypnotherapist. Even now I talk/listen to myself when alone on a regular basis – to check how I sound. I rehearse before making a recording for a client and I listen back to what I have recorded. I am constantly reminding myself about tone, pitch, emphasis, pace, pauses and silences.

A student needs to do the same thing i.e. practise reading scripts out loud – when they are alone, with other students and eventually with real clients. This book is full of scripts to help them with this.

### Training schools

Trainers who deliver hypnotherapy courses need to have resources which they can utilise with students when delivering training classes (face-to-face or online) and which they can recommend for students to read/use. Although regrets are a specialised subject, the scripts in the book can be used for everyday practise as discussed above and explained more in the following chapter.

### Qualified and experienced hypnotherapists

If a hypnotherapist likes to use scripts, then it is useful to have a book which is full of them. It is always good to work with new, fresh materials so that you do not become stale or complacent.

### Supervisors

Practitioners must cover the four functions of supervision in any supervision session (i.e. management; support; education and mediation) and consequently there can be many tasks to perform in the role of supervisor. It is essential that a supervisor has knowledge and skills, but they also need to keep up-to-date and have fresh materials to recommend to their supervisees.

## Road of regrets and stages of the process

Throughout the book I refer to the *road of regrets*, which is discussed more fully in Chapter 10. The road of regrets is a concept I have developed over the years for clients to work with when working through their regrets. The road is travelled during hypnotherapy sessions and the aim is to reach the final destination i.e. living life without the regrets. The road helps the client to understand that regrets are a normal part of everyday life, but there is a need to do some work on the significant ones and the associated emotions whilst travelling along the road. The client is likely to meet obstacles and roadworks along the way, they may be diverted or choose to go in a different direction. In developing the concept of the road of regrets, I have also developed a process, which includes five stages, to give structure to a treatment plan:

• Identifying and acknowledging regrets (Stage 1)
• Working through regrets by looking back at the past and considering what happened; and identifying the associated emotions (Stage 2)
• Taking action(s) to deal with any unresolved issues (Stage 3)

- Releasing the regrets and emotions (Stage 4)
- Planning for the future (Stage 5).

I believe that a properly qualified hypnotherapist should have the skills to help a client through all five stages. A point I want to make and emphasise (and another reason I believe this book is needed) is that taking action (Stage 3) is a really important part of the process. The hypnotherapist needs to discuss with the client whether some sort of action needs to be taken; and if so to support the client whilst that is done. I say frequently to clients: "You cannot change the past but you can change the way you think and feel about it" because this is central to the therapeutic process. So although we cannot change what has happened already, there are some situations where the client could do something in order to help the regrets diminish; many clients say "I need to put things right". Dealing with regrets is not just about identifying the regrets and then planning for the future. In between those stages of the process, some practical action may be needed and may also take some considerable time. It is often said that hypnotherapy is a quick therapy compared to other therapies. However, when working with regrets it may take longer, i.e. more sessions are needed than when working on other issues and could spread out over a longer period of time.

I have already explained that I work as both an independent social worker and a hypnotherapist; and sometimes I am acting in both roles with a client. Over the decades I have undertaken many different tasks in order to support a client. Many of the tasks have involved finding out what happened in the past. Things I have done regularly have been to discover:

- What happened to a baby who was given up for adoption or a baby that was "given away". A typical example being where an adult with learning disabilities was locked away in a mental institution years ago because she had got pregnant and the baby was taken away immediately after the birth.
- How somebody died
- Where a baby/child/adult was cremated/buried
- An actual person e.g. a father who was never known; a relative/friend/colleague who disappeared.

I have convened and mediated meetings between a client and someone they needed to meet/confront. Some hypnotherapists may feel it is not their role to actually get involved in doing research on behalf of a client and I totally understand that. Nevertheless, it is important to help the client identify what action needs to be taken and the hypnotherapist can support the client emotionally whilst the client does the research and then does whatever they need to do themselves.

Whatever action is needed to plan for the future will be different for each client, because their circumstances and situations will vary. The role of the hypnotherapist is to help the client identify what action needs to be taken; and some of this may involve facing the past. Facing the past could involve the client meeting with a person or people to:

- Explain their own actions (or inaction) i.e. why they did or said something (or why they did not say or do something)
- Find out why a person acted as they did
- Find out the truth: what really did happen
- Say sorry
- Make amends.

Once any action which is needed has been completed, then the client can work through Stages 4 and 5 to release the emotions and regrets and ultimately move towards their future without regrets.

## Travelling around the book

Through the different parts of the book, the hypnotherapist will find scripts which facilitate using different modes of transport whilst on the road of regrets. However, it often happens that the client will choose a unique way of travelling for themselves. In order to help the hypnotherapist to quickly find appropriate scripts and visualisations to use with their clients, the following chapter explains how the book is laid out and includes a guide to each chapter and the purpose of each script.

## Note

1 Pritchard, J. (2022) *Dealing with Different Types of Losses Using Hypnotherapy Scripts.* Abingdon, Oxon: Routledge

# Chapter 2

# How to use the book

## Introduction

The book is full of scripts which have a range of objectives and can be used to deal with various types of regrets and their associated emotions. Therefore, it is imperative that a hypnotherapist can find their way around the book easily and not have to spend ages looking for what they need. Obviously, the contents and index can be used, but the purpose of this chapter is to briefly explain how the book is laid out, how it has been divided up into eight parts and then to include a guide to the chapters and scripts. Scripts have been included for both adults and children (age 5+).

## The layout

The first six chapters of the book are full of theoretical discussion and follow the normal format of a chapter as you would expect. For the rest of the book most chapters start with the heading *Introduction*, which will explain the purpose and content of the chapter and stimulate ideas for practice. Each chapter contains one or more scripts and some will have appendices, which serve different purposes. Some appendices include questions or questionnaires, checklists, summaries, forms (which have been included for note-taking/recording purposes), and worksheets for exercises.

The scripts within chapters are of varying length and some short additional scripts are included in some chapters. Within the scripts there are *guidance notes* for the hypnotherapist where needed. I have not written within the scripts words which need emphasis or where pauses or silences should occur. The hypnotherapist needs to work with and respond to the client during a session i.e. work in a person-centred way and go at their pace. Instead *guidance notes* are included within the body of the scripts and at points suggested prompts and/or questions are given, which the hypnotherapist can choose to use or not.

DOI: 10.4324/9781003468325-3

## Using the scripts: preparation

Some scripts were originally written for children. However, many of the scripts which were written for adults can be adapted to be used with a child/young person if the language is changed. It can also work the other way round too; some scripts written for young people can work well for adults with amendments.

The hypnotherapist should always prepare for using a script by:

- Reading the script several times in order to become familiar with it.
- Making any written amendments to the script to suit the needs of the client. This could include making it age appropriate to the client by changing the language.
- Deciding if the script will be used in conjunction with another script or visualisation.
- Making notes on the script and/or including their own: questions; prompts; direct/indirect statements; suggestions; commands which need to be embedded; endings (e.g. ego boosting).
- Rehearsing the script with the aim to present it in their own way i.e. reading the script out loud a number of times. After rehearsing a script and having heard how it sounds, the hypnotherapist may make further amendments to the language and/or add to their notes. The hypnotherapist should keep rehearsing until the script feels and sounds right.
- Timing how long it takes to read the script and allowing enough time for interaction with the client (although this can be difficult to predict accurately in advance of a session). An essential part of preparation is planning sufficient time for a session. A client should never be rushed nor should a session be brought to an abrupt end because the hypnotherapist has another client booked in or they have to get out of the therapy room if the therapy room is hired and needed by another therapist.
- Thinking about the use of their:
  - Voice
  - Tone
  - Pitch
  - Emphasis
  - Pace
  - Pauses
  - Silences.

  It can be really useful for students and newly qualified hypnotherapists to record themselves (using a phone or dictaphone) as they are rehearsing and then listen back to the recording.
- Being aware of their own body language: how they are sitting and what their body does as they read the script out loud.

## Advice for students

When training to become a hypnotherapist, a student will be learning lots of different things regarding theory, methods and techniques; and hopefully will have lots of opportunities to put the theory into practice as they learn in the classroom. Role play is particularly essential to practise good presentation, listening and responding skills, including the things already mentioned above regarding how to speak. Before using scripts, it is imperative for a student to be taught about abreactions and how to handle them. An abreaction is when the subconscious mind brings forward a memory and the client relives a traumatic event from the past. When this happens spontaneously, it can sometimes be very scary for the both the client and the hypnotherapist. On occasions a client can become abusive and/or violent. It is important that the hypnotherapist remains calm; and ideally the abreaction should not be stopped unless a person is at risk of harm (which could be the client, the hypnotherapist or both of them). The client should be encouraged to stay with the memory and relive the event/experience through to the end. Therefore, it is vital that a student is taught which techniques can be useful in these situations and to have plenty of practise role playing different scenarios.

## Process and parts

In the previous chapter I introduced the concept of the *road of regrets* and explained that I have developed a structure to work through the regrets, which includes five stages:

- Identifying and acknowledging regrets (Stage 1)
- Working through regrets by looking back at the past and considering what happened; and identifying the associated emotions (Stage 2)
- Taking action(s) to deal with any unresolved issues (Stage 3)
- Releasing the regrets and emotions (Stage 4)
- Planning for the future (Stage 5).

The book is structured to follow the process but has additional parts as explained below.

## The parts

What follows is a brief summary of what each part contains in the book.

### I  Working with regrets

This part initially introduces the book by discussing the important subject of regrets and its relevance to the work of the hypnotherapist. Different types of regrets are then discussed in more detail, followed by a chapter about the emotions associated with regrets. Next, attention is given to the importance of undertaking thorough assessments; followed by a chapter which focuses on how groupwork can be an effective way of working with regrets.

## II   Scripts for the first session

Three scripts are presented in this part, which can be used to introduce the client to hypnosis and the trance state. Two of the scripts are aimed at clients who may be either auditory or olfactory.

## III   Identifying and acknowledging regrets

The concept of the *road of regrets*, which is revisited throughout the book, is introduced and explained. It is important for the hypnotherapist to have a clear understanding of this and how it can be used with a client who will travel along the road. Right at the beginning of the process (Stage 1) time must be spent identifying and acknowledging the client's regrets. The scripts in this part facilitate this.

## IV   Working through emotions

So many emotions can be associated with regrets and the hypnotherapist will always be considering a client's thoughts, feelings and behaviours. There are many different methods and techniques which can be used to help the client work on their emotions (Stage 2). The scripts will help the client to talk about how they feel about the regrets – both from the past and in the present. Several of the scripts include regression techniques, so that the root cause of a regret can be worked with in one or more sessions.

## V   Taking action

Some of the work to be undertaken with a client can involve helping them to take some practical action in regard to their regrets e.g. meeting with/confronting someone (Stage 3), but this can be very scary for some people. Planning, preparation and rehearsal are essential to do this successfully. Anyone who enjoys using Gestalt techniques will find some useful scripts here. The client looks at how they present themselves and also becomes aware of other people's body language and behaviour in various situations.

## VI   Releasing

Stage 4 of the process is about releasing the regrets and the emotions (i.e. thoughts and feelings) associated with them. The scripts in this part offer many different ways of doing this and they continue the theme of being able to move in different ways along the road of regrets.

## VII    Planning for the future

The scripts in this part should be used once all the regrets have been released and the client is ready to plan for their future living without regrets (Stage 5).

## VIII    Additional scripts

The previous sections include scripts which are specific to the particular stage of the process they are concerned with. However, I have written scripts which can be used in several stages of the process; such scripts are included in this part. Several metaphorical scripts are also included.

## Guide to the chapters/scripts

The guide should be used to find an appropriate script/subject area.

1.  Introduction: why we should work with regrets
    *Why regrets need to be given attention and the book is needed. Explains the objectives of the book and who will find the book useful. Introduces the concept of the road of regrets and the stages of the process.*
2.  How to use the book
    *Explains how the book is set out in parts and what is included. A guide to the scripts – and what they can be used for.*
3.  Different types of regrets
    *Lays the foundations for thinking about the different types of regrets which a hypnotherapist may have to work with. Discusses in full the grouping of regrets used in the book.*
4.  Emotions associated with regrets
    *Discusses and defines emotions. Considers the link between thoughts, feelings and behaviours. Includes two exercises.*
    *Appendix 4.1: Negative emotions and feelings associated with regrets*
    *Appendix 4.2: Positive emotions and feelings having worked through regrets*
    *Appendix 4.3: Worksheet for Exercise 4.1 – Focusing on emotions*
    *Appendix 4.4: Worksheet for Exercise 4.2 – A regret, thoughts, feelings and behaviours*
    *Appendix 4.5: Form for recording thoughts, feelings and behaviours*
5.  Assessment for regrets
    *Discusses the importance of assessment before and during the first session. Identifying regrets. Mind mapping. Failing and failures. The benefits approach.*
    *Script: To identify regrets. For when the client is already working on a problem, but has not mentioned the word "regret" however the hypnotherapist thinks there are regrets to be identified.*

15. Pathways through the woods

    *To regress the client using pathways through the woods. Can be used in several sessions if necessary.*

    *Ending: The picnic basket. Can be used to terminate the script; to plan action or to look to the future.*

16. The square to the past

    *To regress the client either to earlier in their current life or a past life.*

17. Russian dolls

    *For the client to look at different versions of their self using Russian dolls. Regression technique. Brings forward regrets from the past and current regrets. Plans work to be done.*

    *Appendix 17.1: Form for regrets identified using the Russian dolls*

    *Appendix 17.2: Form for identifying work to be done*

18. Under the microscope

    *The client takes a close look at their thoughts, feelings and behaviours in relation to their regrets.*

19. Walking in the rain

    *Identifies regrets. Works on certain emotions – heaviness; stickiness; being glued together; stuck. Embeds the idea of weathering the storm.*

20. The donkey with a heavy load

    *To work on the feelings when carrying a burden. Heaviness. Tiredness. Exhaustion. Pain – physical or emotional. Focuses on embedding strength; determination; endurance.*

21. Feeling trapped

    *Uses a prison cell to deal with the feelings of being trapped. No way out. Uses the imagination as a distraction/escape and to stop intrusive thoughts. To break free.*

22. Stuck, frozen and numb

    *To deal with these specific feelings.*

    *Script 1: Stuck in the snow. Focuses on being stuck. Feeling frozen. Finding the way out and going forward.*

    *Script 2: Being at the dentist. Considers the benefits of numbness to avoid pain. To experience new sensations.*

23. Why I did what I did

    *To understand the thoughts and feelings underpinning the client's behaviour.*

24. I should have

    *For the client to reflect back on what they regret having done. Then to plan any action for the future.*

    *Appendix 24.1: Form for identifying the "I should have's"*

    *Appendix 24.2: Form for actions to be taken*

25. Fear of failing

*For a child or adult to understand that failures are a normal part of life and lessons can be learnt from them. To change the way of thinking and feeling about failing and failures. To work on building confidence and self-esteem.*

*Appendix 25.1: Form for recording failings and failures identified*

26. Street art

*For clients who find it difficult to talk verbally or express their emotions. Promotes expression through artwork and using electricity power cabinets. Emphasises being in control; being able to turn things on and off; having power and surging.*

27. Let's think about the Rs

*For reflecting on and reviewing the regrets already identified.*

28. It's never too late

*For use when a client is going to plan some action in relation to their regrets.*

*Additional script: Optional mantra. Can be used to develop a mantra.*

29. The meeting room

*A meeting room is set up for the client to plan, prepare and rehearse a situation, conversation or confrontation.*

*Additional script: Confrontation can be a positive thing*

30. Communication and presenting oneself

*To work on communication skills by looking at body language; body positioning and movement; voice; eye contact; facial expressions and breathing.*

31. Your own channel

*Creating a video to either plan and rehearse a situation or talk about thoughts and feelings.*

*Option 1: Preparing for a meeting/conversation*

*Option 2: The need to talk/vent*

32. I'm sorry

*To get the client to be specific about what they are actually sorry about. To prepare for explaining this to someone else.*

33. The drainage system

*To drain away the regrets using the image of water.*

34. Cliff edge

*To acknowledge the client has been on a hard, steep climb working through their regrets. To throw away the regrets into the sea.*

35. Ice cubes melting

*To dissolve negative feelings. Considers experiencing extreme temperatures.*

36. Bubble machine

*To blow the regrets away. Float into the future. To feel safe. For relaxation.*

37. Army of ants

*To work systematically by having a plan and a strategy to carry regrets away. Feeling upright – steady – and secure.*

38. Flying with the birds

    *To deal with the feelings of being stuck or trapped. To leave the situation which has caused these feelings. Can be used for relaxation purposes in future sessions.*

39. Dusting and hoovering up

    *To dust away the particles (thoughts and feelings) and hoover up trodden in dirt (regrets). To make fresh and clean for the future.*

40. Let's have a declutter

    *To declutter the mind of unnecessary items e.g. thoughts; feelings; behaviours; memories; people. To focus on happiness. To reorganise and tidy up for the future.*

41. Car wash

    *To clean the car outside and inside. To check and maintain parts. To make fit for purpose. To wash away regrets, thoughts and feelings.*

42. Parking the regrets

    *To pack up, drive, park and leave the regrets behind forever.*

43. Visualisations for breaking free and cutting off

    *To cut loose from negative emotions/the feelings and cutting off associated with the regrets.*

    *The script: general introduction for visualisations*
    1. *Air raid shelter*
    2. *Tied up at the docks*
    3. *Chopping vegetables.*

44. The world is your oyster

    *To identify what the client wants in the future (the pearl). To embed positivity for the future.*

45. It's my life

    *For clients who regret putting the needs of others before themselves. To address feelings of guilt. To focus on themselves: needs; wishes; hopes; aspirations; ambitions.*

    *Additional script 1: To remember the past*
    *Additional script 2: The mantra – It's my life*

46. Drawing and crossing a line

    *To leave regrets behind the line drawn. To cross the line into the future.*
    *The script: General introduction*
    *Additional script 1: On the beach*
    *Additional script 2: On the road*

47. Galloping and racing into the future

    *Preparing to enter a race into the future. Works on motivation and determination. Promotes the idea of strength in both body and mind.*

48. Designing a magazine cover

    *The client considers how they want to be in the future and who they want to have in their life. Promotes a positive image, which conveys messages for the readership i.e. people the client wants to have in their life.*

49. Stained glass windows

    *To design windows to tell the story of the client's future.*

50. Freya the fox and the eggs

    *Metaphor for a child to address the feelings of guilt when they have done something which they did not know was wrong. Demonstrates how to say or show you are sorry.*

51. Sophia the seamstress

    *Metaphor. To work on feelings of guilt resulting from not having been able to protect someone. Focuses on domestic abuse. Sophia develops coping strategies in childhood and adulthood.*

52. Not having a childhood

    *Young carers: discussion/statistics. Followed by metaphor. For young carers. For adults who feel they did not have a childhood. Living in poverty. Regrets about stealing, being violent. Conflicted emotions about people/relationships: love; care; loyalty; duty; responsibility; hate; anger and resentment.*

53. On the motorway

    *To work with the concept of the road of regrets. Can be used at different stages of the process. Facilitates one or more journeys. Final drive away from the regrets.*

54. Rowing

    *An alternative mode of transport to travel the road of regrets. To build strength and determination. Can be used more than once at various stages of the process. Or use just once to get to the final destination on the road of regrets.*

    *Additional script 1: Rowing to regress. Rowing back in time to a significant event which has caused the regrets.*

55. The computer screen

    *To focus on regrets, thoughts and feelings by creating pages. Looks at self via the webcam. Creates pages related to the past (and deletes them). Creates pages for the future (and saves them). Changes are seen via the webcam.*

56. High wire act

    *To work on performance. For clients who lack confidence; do not think they are good enough; have regrets about not studying; not training; not being ambitious.*

# Chapter 3

# Different types of regrets

Everyone has regrets and they will occur at different points throughout a lifetime. Every day a person will experience some minor regret, which is not going to have a major impact on their life; for example, regretting that you have worn the new shoes you have on today because your feet are really hurting. Regrets which are trivial or minor are unlikely to have a great or noticeable impact on you and are probably quickly forgotten. Some regrets are more serious. A regret can play on a person's mind for a while and then it seems to fade away; however, at a certain point in life the regret can come forward again and then does not go away. The resurrection of a regret can be caused by any number of things – reaching a certain milestone, an event, an incident, a crisis or some kind a change. Typical examples are:

*   Major birthdays e.g. 18, 21, 30, 40, 50, 60
*   Becoming a parent
*   Menopause
*   Being made redundant
*   Retirement
*   Failing to get a job/position because of not having the right qualifications
*   When something comes to an end (e.g. school, college, university; relationship; marriage; friendship)
*   When diagnosed with a health problem/terminal illness
*   Experiencing a loss/death/bereavement
*   When someone comes back into a person's life.

Occasionally, it is not any of the above situations that cause regrets to occur. Rather a person simply realises that time is precious and it passes very quickly; therefore, you should make the most of life. It is never too late to do the things you want to do.

Certain regrets may seem unimportant, but the fact that they occasionally enter one's mind indicates they are of some significance. Other regrets may start to regularly come into the conscious mind and may also be the subject of recurring dreams. A person can begin to think about their regrets so frequently it becomes obsessive. Clients can describe these types of regrets as "eating away at me" or they say "I just

DOI: 10.4324/9781003468325-4

can't stop thinking about [*regret*]". If these regrets continue they can eventually have a massive impact on a person's life, which is why they need appropriate help, support and therapy. I believe a hypnotherapist can be the ideal person to provide this if the client is willing to work on the regrets and make changes in their life.

I do not think it is a regular occurrence for a person to seek help specifically for the regrets they are experiencing. A person may be feeling a certain way (e.g. lethargic; not motivated; low-mood; depressed; anxious) and in the conscious state is not realising what is causing these feelings. Consequently, the regrets may be brought forward as the hypnotherapist works with the client. As has already been mentioned in Chapter 1, I believe it is imperative to work with the regrets and not dismiss them. But what types of regrets may a hypnotherapist have to work with through a treatment plan? Before considering this further it may be helpful to define a regret. A person can feel regret or be regretful, but the therapy needs to focus on the actual regret. This can often be difficult for the client to define and hence why using hypnosis can be so effective, i.e. working with the subconscious mind to identify what the actual regret is.

## Some dictionary definitions of regrets

When giving consideration to a specific subject I think it can be thought-provoking and valuable for reflection purposes to consider definitions from dictionaries. Regrets are defined as follows:

> a feeling of sadness, repentance, or disappointment over an occurrence or something that one has done or failed to do
>
> (Oxford Learners)[1]

> a feeling of sadness about something sad or wrong or about a mistake that you have made, and a wish that it could have been different and better
>
> (Cambridge English Dictionary)[2]

> sorrow aroused by circumstances beyond one's control or power to repair
> an expression of distressing emotion (such as sorrow)
>
> (Merriam-Webster)[3]

> A feeling of sorrow, disappointment, distress, or remorse about something that one wishes could be different.
>
> (The Free Dictionary)[4]

> A sense of loss and longing for someone or something gone or passed out of existence
> a sense of loss, disappointment, dissatisfaction, etc.
> a feeling of sorrow or remorse for a fault, act, loss, disappointment, etc
>
> (Dictionary.com)[5]

## Grouping the regrets

It would be impossible (and it is not the purpose) to consider in this book every single regret a person could experience. However, it is important and helpful to initially think about the different types of regrets which might be presented to a hypnotherapist and give some examples. A vital stage of the process (Stage 1) in working with regrets is for the hypnotherapist to help the client to acknowledge and identify the regrets. You often hear people say they regret what they have not done rather than what they have done. This is usually in regard to a missed opportunity and maybe they feel it is too late to do anything about it (Chapter 28 presents a script to address this).

There are times in our lives when we just fall into a way of being and doing. We do not consciously make a decision; we just get on with life. However, as time goes on a person may look back and regret how they lived their life at a certain point in time. A typical example is someone who did not enjoy school for whatever reason and did not take learning very seriously. Or they were just having a good social life, stayed out late every night and did not study nor revise. Years later the regret may be that they did not achieve any qualifications and they have not enjoyed the jobs/ career path they have followed. Other regrets can relate to more conscious decisions made e.g. choosing not to stay on at school or go to college; rather to go and get a job; or choosing to go to live in a particular place for university, a job or to be in a relationship. A person can regret the lifestyle choice they have consciously made or they have fallen into because of peer group pressure e.g. running with a gang; using drugs. It is important to acknowledge that sometimes a person does not have a choice and they are powerless, because they are being made to do something by someone else who is in control i.e. with the power.

Consequently, it can be helpful to put regrets into some basic groupings:

*   Choices/decisions
*   Missed opportunities
*   Things done
*   Things not done
*   Things said
*   Things not said.

All of the groupings above could relate to oneself or others. More specific groupings can be developed to think about subject areas that a regret may be related to; some examples being:

*   Actions
*   Inaction
*   Behaviours
*   Relationships
*   Experiences

- Work/career
- Hobbies/leisure/travel
- Learning/studying/training/skills/knowledge.

What follows are some typical examples in relation to the basic groupings, but obviously these lists are not exhaustive and the reader might like to try to add examples from their own personal and work experiences:

### Choices/decisions made/missed opportunities:

- Not studying
- Not learning
- Skiving from school
- Subjects chosen for GCSEs; A Levels; Degree
- Not staying on at school
- College/university: going/not going; where/location
- Learning a skill/trade
- Taking a certain career path
- Not pursuing hobbies
- Places to see/go.

### Things done (or said):

- Lying/not being honest/omitting the truth
- Cheating (e.g. in a relationship; in exams; getting someone to write an essay; plagiarism)
- Bullying
- Abusing
- Harming/hurting someone (e.g. physically; psychologically; neglect)
- Killing someone (accidentally or pre-meditated)
- Forcing someone to do something
- Excessive spending (perhaps resulting in bankruptcy)
- Drinking excessively (alcoholism)
- Taking drugs (long-term effects being illness; mental health issues)
- Gambling
- Eating unhealthily
- Following a particular lifestyle (e.g. being in a gang)
- Committing a crime
- Fraud/theft
- Falsifying documents
- Sleeping around; spreading a sexually transmitted disease
- Being jealous/envious
- Being in a particular relationship
- Having an abortion

- Giving a baby/child up for adoption
- Getting married
- Getting divorced
- Controlling someone or a situation
- Being too strict (as a parent)
- Being a carer
- Putting career on hold
- Following other people's wishes
- Following cultural or religious traditions (e.g. agreeing to an arranged marriage)
- Succumbing to peer pressure.

### Things not done (or said):

- Something earlier in life
- Asking questions when you had the chance (e.g. when a person was still alive)
- Standing up to someone
- Standing up for self/others
- Speaking out/saying something (e.g. about a colleague; work situation; stealing ideas/work)
- Protecting someone
- Telling/disclosing (e.g. about an abuser/abusive situation)
- Confronting someone
- Leaving a situation (home; relationship; job)
- Following your heart (doing sensible thing; always taking the safe pathway; listened to others rather than self)
- Having a relationship/friendship (with someone who has particular qualities/ personality/characteristics/interests; with a particular person)
- Attending an event (birth; school event; graduation; wedding; funeral)
- Being a good partner/parent/friend/colleague
- Spending enough time with ... (child; parent; friend)
- Having children
- Having more children
- Having a particular conversation
- Expressing emotional feelings (saying how you feel; how something felt)
- Supporting someone (physically, emotionally or financially)
- Saying goodbye
- Attempting/having a go (activity; job)
- Taking medication
- Having treatment
- Facing reality (being in denial)
- Tackling/confronting discrimination
- Coming out (earlier)
- Following a particular career/job

- Learning a trade/skill
- Going for promotion
- Being ambitious
- Looking for someone
- Finding out the truth.

## Failing and failure

Some therapists do not think we should dwell on failing and failures. However, it is a fact we all fail at things (e.g. remembering when someone's birthday is; an exam; driving test) and hopefully learn from those failures. Regrets can often link to a person believing they have failed themselves or others. So identifying the failures and learning from them may be necessary to work through the regrets. In Chapter 5, failing and failures are discussed in relation to the assessment process and Chapter 25 addresses the fear of failing.

## Self-reflection and the hypnotherapist

When training to become a hypnotherapist, a person should be undertaking a lot of self-analysis with support from their trainer. Any therapist or worker in the caring professions needs to work on themselves and deal with any unresolved issues/problems in their own life. This is important when training but once qualified the hypnotherapist should regularly undertake self-reflection in order to continue to develop both personally and professionally and to practise safely. This can be undertaken in supervision sessions and in addition the hypnotherapist might also want to reflect on their practice for the purpose of continuing professional development (CPD). Whilst reading through this book a hypnotherapist might want to undertake a reflective exercise to identify their own regrets and failures. To summarise the hypnotherapist should reflect on:

- Their own regrets
- Regrets in personal life
- Regrets which are work-related
- The timing of the regrets
- Their own thoughts, feelings and behaviours
- Working with clients on regrets
- Work they have done; what worked and what did not work; what they have learnt from this
- Work they would like to do on regrets in the future.

The hypnotherapist could also use the exercises and appendices in other chapters to evidence that they have done this. In order to work through regrets work has to be done on the associated emotions. The following chapter considers this subject and again the hypnotherapist might wish to do think about emotions in relation to their own regrets.

## Notes

1 https://www.oxfordlearnersdictionaries.com/definition/english/regret_1
2 https://dictionary.cambridge.org/dictionary/english/regret
3 https://www.merriam-webster.com/dictionary/regret
4 https://www.thefreedictionary.com/regret
5 https://www.dictionary.com/browse/regret (Accessed April 2024)

Chapter 4

# Emotions associated with regrets

Emotions are a reaction to stimuli. They are the result of how we react to something, someone or a situation we find ourselves in. Having regrets can result in experiencing certain emotions – more often negative rather than positive emotions. Feelings are what we experience as a result of an emotion and can be longer lasting. Hypnotherapists spend a lot of time working with thoughts, feelings and behaviours. The three things are interconnected and I always spend a considerable amount of time talking to my clients about this, because it helps them understand the interaction and what we are working towards i.e. to facilitate change. It is beneficial for a client to consider how their thoughts can influence their feelings; how their feelings can influence their thoughts; and how both thoughts and feelings can influence their behaviour.

When developing a treatment plan the hypnotherapist and the client need to consider what changes the client needs to work on. The way a person thinks, feels and behaves can become a habit, which in turn can be detrimental to their wellbeing. It is useful to remember that both physical health and mental health contribute to one's wellbeing; and experiencing ongoing negative emotions can adversely affect one's mental health. When a person has regrets they may experience a whole gamut of emotions; and these can change over time. If the regrets are not dealt with they can become overwhelming, all-consuming and dominate a person's life i.e. their thoughts, feelings and behaviours. This can result in obsessive thought patterns and behaviours.

## Some dictionary definitions of an emotion

As already stated in the previous chapter it can be useful to consider the meaning of words by looking at some dictionary definitions. An emotion is defined as:

a strong feeling deriving from one's circumstances, mood, or relationships with others

DOI: 10.4324/9781003468325-5

a strong feeling such as love, fear or anger; the part of a person's character that consists of feelings

(Oxford Learners)[1]

a strong feeling such as love or anger, or strong feelings in general

(Cambridge English Dictionary)[2]

an emotion is a feeling such as happiness, love, fear, anger, or hatred, which can be caused by the situation that you are in or the people you are with

(Collins Dictionary)[3]

a: conscious mental reaction (such as anger or fear) subjectively experienced as strong feeling usually directed toward a specific object and typically accompanied by physiological and behavioural changes in the body

b: a state of feeling

c: the affective aspect of consciousness: **FEELING**

(Merriam Webster)[4]

an affective state of consciousness in which joy, sorrow, fear, hate, or the like, is experienced, as distinguished from cognitive and volitional states of consciousness

(Dictionary.com)[5]

A mental state that arises spontaneously rather than through conscious effort and is often accompanied by physiological changes; a feeling: *the emotions of joy, sorrow, and anger*
Such mental states or the qualities that are associated with them, especially in contrast to reason: *a decision based on emotion rather than logic*

(The Free Dictionary)[6]

Below is a list of negative emotions and feelings, which I have compiled from the actual words used by clients when working through their regrets and the emotions; and are not in any particular order of priority or frequency used. This list is also presented in Appendix 4.1, so that the hypnotherapist can use it as a checklist; or it can also be used as handout for discussion with a client or for a student hypnotherapist with their trainer or supervisor:

- Sad
- Upset
- Lost
- Alone
- Lonely
- Isolated
- Detached
- Low
- Depressed
- Abandoned
- Cut off
- Deserted
- Disassociated
- Despondent
- Despair
- Pessimistic
- Anxious
- Scared
- Fearful
- Panic
- Overwhelmed
- Stuck
- Trapped
- Hemmed in
- Claustrophobic
- Restricted
- Unable to move freely
- Tied up
- Held back
- Unconfident
- Weak
- Stupid
- Angry
- Furious
- Bitter
- Resentful
- Hatred
- Deprived
- Missed out
- Vengeful
- Obligated
- Dutiful
- Duty bound
- Responsible
- Guilt
- Blame
- Self-blame
- Jealous
- Let down
- Cheated
- Betrayed
- Mistrustful
- Distrustful
- Wary
- Doubtful
- Suspicious
- Frustrated
- Failed
- A failure
- Failing
- Numb
- Useless
- Hopeless
- Helpless
- Worthless
- Shame
- Intimidated
- Degraded
- Humiliated
- Embarrassed
- Redundant
- Purposeless
- Directionless
- Powerless
- Out of control
- Paranoid
- Bogged down
- Dragged down
- Immobile
- Burdened
- Numb
- Frozen
- Cold
- Hardened
- Drained
- Tired
- Exhausted
- Pain

It is very easy just to focus on the negative emotions and feelings. I think it is equally important to give attention to the positive emotions and feelings a client may experience when they have reached the end of the process (the final destination on their road of regrets). Clients can feel they have learnt from their regrets and having those experiences. A client may talk about this naturally in the last few sessions, but some hypnotherapists will want to evaluate more formally the work which has been undertaken with the client. This is often done verbally but some hypnotherapists will develop an evaluation form which they ask the client to complete after the last session; and sometimes again 3 or 6 months later for further feedback and evaluation after time for reflection.

Another list is presented below using the actual words of clients again regarding positive emotions and feelings they have experienced having travelled along the road of regrets and reached their final destination. This list is presented again in Appendix 4.2:

- Pleased
- Glad
- Happy
- Thankful
- Relieved
- Enlightened
- Unburdened
- Free
- Hopeful
- Optimistic
- Confident
- Excited
- Supported
- Educated
- Motivated
- Determined
- Strong
- Assertive

Negative emotions associated with regrets can result in long-term problematic behaviours, which a hypnotherapist may be dealing with on a daily basis i.e. they are issues not just related to regrets. The common ones being:

- Lack of confidence
- Lack of belief in oneself
- Low self-esteem
- Habits
- Obsessive thoughts
- Obsessive behaviours
- Anxiety
- Panic/panic attacks
- Poor sleep/insomnia
- Trust issues

## Exercises

I like my hypnotherapy sessions to include a variety of activities, one of which is the use of exercises, which can be done with the client in the conscious state and sometimes in the trance state if appropriate. Clients can be very nervous in the first session (and even in the second session sometimes) because they know they are going to have to face some difficult things emotionally. Some clients may also find it difficult to talk because they are shy or lack confidence. So introducing exercises, which involve writing or drawing, can help.

The following two simple exercises can be used to start the client thinking about their emotions and to introduce the idea of thoughts, feelings and behaviours and the link between them. These two exercises can be used in one session i.e. back-to-back; or Exercise 4.1 could be used in an early session and then Exercise 4.2 in the following session to go into more detail about the link between thoughts, feelings and behaviours and undertake more in-depth work.

Appendices 4.3 and 4.4 include worksheets for the client to use. These exercises can also be used in a regrets groups (see Chapter 6) or be given as "homework" to do in between sessions.

### Exercise 4.1: Focusing on emotions

**Purpose of the exercise**: to get the client to think about the emotions they have experienced earlier in the day and then to focus on one simple one in order to introduce the idea of thoughts, feelings and behaviours and the link between them.

**Equipment needed**: Appendix 4.3; worksheet and pens.

The hypnotherapist should explain the purpose of the exercise and go through the questions which are listed on the worksheet:

1. Think about what you have been doing today: where you have been; things you have done; people you have met.
2. Make a list of the emotions (using only one word) you have experienced during the course of the day.
3. Pick one emotion from the list above. Make a list of any thoughts you had whilst experiencing this emotion.
4. Describe any of the feelings (use as many words as you like) you had when experiencing this emotion.
5. Did your behaviour change in any way at this time? If yes, how did it change?

The client is then left to think and write on the worksheet. I usually allocate up to ten minutes for this activity. Once the client has completed the task the hypnotherapist will initiate a full discussion by asking the client to talk about what they have written on the worksheet.

### Exercise 4.2: A regret, thoughts, feelings and behaviours

**Purpose of the exercise**: to facilitate the client to focus on one specific regret and then to identify the thoughts, feelings and behaviours associated with that regret.

**Equipment needed**: Appendix 4.4; worksheet and pens.

The hypnotherapist should explain the purpose of the exercise and go through the questions which are listed on the worksheet:

1. The regret: think about one of the regrets you have.
2. Thoughts: What comes into your head when you think about the regret?
3. Feelings: What are you feeling now as you are thinking about the regret?
4. Behaviours: Has this regret affected/changed your behaviour in anyway? If yes, how?

As in the previous exercise, the client is then left to think and write on the worksheet for up to ten minutes and then a full discussion will take place.

## Emotions in the process of working through regrets

Talking about emotions and feelings is going to be a crucial part of any hypnotherapy session whatever the issue/problem being worked on in a treatment plan. It will be no different when working through regrets. However, there will be greater emphasis on addressing emotions during Stage 2 of the process, when the associated emotions will be identified; and Stage 4 when the emotions are released. In Appendix 4.5 I have included a form which can be used at any stage of the process for the hypnotherapist to be able to record a regret and the related thoughts, feelings and behaviours.

## Appendix 4.1: Negative emotions and feelings associated with regrets

- Sad
- Upset
- Lost
- Alone
- Lonely
- Isolated
- Detached
- Low
- Depressed
- Abandoned
- Cut off
- Deserted
- Disassociated
- Despondent
- Despair
- Pessimistic
- Anxious
- Scared
- Fearful
- Panic
- Overwhelmed
- Stuck
- Trapped
- Hemmed in
- Claustrophobic
- Restricted
- Unable to move freely
- Tied up
- Held back
- Unconfident
- Weak
- Stupid
- Angry
- Furious
- Bitter
- Resentful
- Hatred
- Deprived
- Missed out
- Vengeful
- Obligated
- Dutiful
- Duty bound
- Responsible

- Guilt
- Blame
- Self-blame
- Jealous
- Let down
- Cheated
- Betrayed
- Mistrustful
- Distrustful
- Wary
- Doubtful
- Suspicious
- Frustrated
- Failed
- A failure
- Failing
- Numb
- Useless
- Hopeless
- Helpless
- Worthless
- Shame
- Intimidated
- Degraded
- Humiliated
- Embarrassed
- Redundant
- Purposeless
- Directionless
- Powerless
- Out of control
- Paranoid
- Bogged down
- Dragged down
- Immobile
- Burdened
- Numb
- Frozen
- Cold
- Hardened
- Drained
- Tired
- Exhausted
- Pain

## Appendix 4.2: Positive emotions and feelings having worked through the regrets

- Pleased
- Glad
- Happy
- Thankful
- Relieved
- Enlightened
- Unburdened
- Free
- Hopeful
- Optimistic
- Confident
- Excited
- Supported
- Educated
- Motivated
- Determined
- Strong
- Assertive

## Appendix 4.3: Worksheet for Exercise 4.1 – Focusing on emotions

### *FOCUSING ON EMOTIONS*

1.   Think about what you have been doing today: where you have been; things you have done; people you have met.

2.   Make a list of the emotions (using only one word) you have experienced during the course of the day.

3.   Pick one emotion from the list above: _____.
     Make a list of any thoughts you had whilst experiencing this emotion.

4.   Describe any of the feelings (use as many words as you like) you had when experiencing this emotion.

5.   Did your behaviour change in any way at this time?

     [ ] Yes          [ ] No

     If yes, how did it change?

**Appendix 4.4: Worksheet for Exercise 4.2 – A regret, thoughts, feelings and behaviours**

### A REGRET, THOUGHTS, FEELINGS AND BEHAVIOURS

1.  The regret: think about one of the regrets you have.

2.  Thoughts: What comes into your head when you think about the regret?

3.  Feelings: What are you feeling now as you are thinking about the regret?

4.  Behaviours: Has this regret affected/changed your behaviour in anyway? If yes, how?

## Appendix 4.5: Form for recording thoughts, feelings and behaviours

### THOUGHTS, FEELINGS AND BEHAVIOURS

Name of client:                                        Date:

**The regret:**

**Thoughts**

**Feelings**

**Behaviour changes over time**

## Notes

1  https://www.oxfordlearnersdictionaries.com/definition/english/emotion?q=emotions
2  https://dictionary.cambridge.org/dictionary/english/emotion
3  https://www.collinsdictionary.com/dictionary/english/emotion#google_vignette
4  https://www.merriam-webster.com/dictionary/emotion
5  https://www.dictionary.com/browse/emotion
6  https://www.thefreedictionary.com/emotion

# Chapter 5

# Assessment for regrets

In any hypnotherapy book I think it is essential to include some discussion about the importance of assessment. Every hypnotherapist should have been trained about the value of thorough assessment procedures. However, I feel I can never emphasise enough how important it is to make sufficient time to assess in depth. It should never be rushed or considered to be something to get through quickly. Extensive notes should be taken about the information given regarding the presenting problem, the client's personal details, history and current situation. In some circumstances, it can be necessary to undertake a further assessment when a new issue/problem arises (i.e. when already working to a treatment plan) and more information is needed about that. This can occur when the hypnotherapist is already working with a client and the subject of regrets comes to the forefront. The hypnotherapist may wish to discuss the subject of regrets with the client in the trance state and then again when back in the conscious state to assess further. It will then be necessary to update/amend the treatment plan.

## Assessment before the first session

The hypnotherapist will have their own way of assessing potential clients. Some offer an assessment by having a conversation on the telephone or online; others will do a full assessment during the first face-to-face session with a client. In my own practice, I like to have a chat on the telephone initially to get some basic information about why the potential client is seeking help. I then talk about hypnosis, how hypnotherapy might help with the problem and then I explain how I work. I explain that if they do book an appointment with me I shall undertake a full assessment during the first session. I also discuss confidentiality and how I store both written and electronic records. I always encourage potential clients to speak to a number of hypnotherapists before deciding who they would like to help them. I also stress that it is vital to check that a hypnotherapist is properly qualified and is registered with one of the professional bodies.

DOI: 10.4324/9781003468325-6

## Assessment during the first session

During a first session I will always spend between 30 and 45 minutes assessing the client; and I do this free of charge. No matter how the hypnotherapist is going to undertake their assessments, the main objective should be to obtain information about the following subjects – some of which may not be relevant to all clients but they still have to be checked out:

- Personal details
- Contact details
- Significant people in personal/work life: family, friends, colleagues
- Any professionals/workers involved
- Physical health: current and past
- Mental health: current and past
- Treatment for conditions
- Medication
- Surgery
- Any current issues/problems (in addition to the presenting problem)
- Counselling/therapy: current and past
- Hypnosis: knowledge; understanding; previous experience
- Fears/phobias
- Hobbies/interests
- Reasons for wanting to try hypnosis/hypnotherapy: objectives; wishes.

I have developed a separate list of questions for use when assessing a client who needs to work on regrets. For a new client I would go through the subjects as listed above and then I would use the additional questions as follows:

1. What regrets do you have?
2. Do these regrets stem back to:
   - Distant past
   - Recent past
   - Childhood
   - Adolescence
   - Adulthood?
3. How often do you think about the regrets?
4. When do you think about the regrets?
5. Is there any particular time you think about them? (*e.g. day; time; anniversary of an event*)
6. Do you dwell on them? If so, for how long at any one time?
7. Do you think regularly about any particular regret? If, so how regularly?
8. When you reflect on your regrets what do you feel?
9. Describe your emotions.

10. Does having these regrets affect your life now? If so, how?
11. Have these regrets affected your life in the past? If so, how?
12. Do you want to do anything in particular in regard to your regrets:
    - Make amends
    - Put things right
    - Find someone
    - Find out the truth
    - Solve a mystery
13. What do you think will gain from working through your regrets? Think about the benefits:
    Benefit 1:
    Benefit 2:
    Benefit 3:
    Benefit 4:
    Benefit 5:

This list of questions is presented in Appendix 5.1 and can be formatted into a questionnaire to send out to potential participants who might be going to attend a regrets group (see the following chapter). If I am already working with a client on a problem and then regrets come up as another issue/problem to be addressed and worked on, I would allocate specific time to undertake a further assessment using this list of questions.

Appendix 5.2 includes a form which can be used for recording the details of the regrets identified in an assessment. The form can also be used in conjunction with scripts from other parts of the books for recording purposes i.e. when regrets are being identified or acknowledged (Stage 2); or when regression techniques are used and regrets come forward from the current life or a past life.

### Assessing and identifying regrets in the conscious state: mind mapping

Some clients find it difficult to verbalise what they are thinking and prefer to write or draw things. This is where mind mapping can help. Appendix 5.3 includes a map which can be used when the client is in the conscious state. It works particularly well with a child as it can be incorporated in the session as a fun activity/game. This should be a fun task for both children and adults. An adult should not see it as a form filling exercise. The client is asked to think about their regrets and then in the circles write a word, a phrase or draw something. It should be emphasised that it is not an expectation that the whole sheet will be filled up; rather the client should use as many circles as they need. The client should be left to do this for five to ten minutes. The hypnotherapist should have a variety of pens, pencils, crayons, felt tip pens etc available to make it more fun. When the map has been completed, discussion will take place about what is visible on the map.

## Talking about failing and failures

In Chapter 3 the concept of failing and failures was mentioned and that we should not shy away from talking about failures, because often good lessons can be learnt from failing. A failure should not be seen solely in terms of being a negative thing. Therefore, when identifying regrets it can be helpful to also work on identifying failures, because regrets and the sense of failing are often inter-linked. This piece of work could be undertaken in the assessment process, but the hypnotherapist may prefer to leave it until a second session when more trust has been built up and established. Hypnotherapists are trained in how to build rapport and will do that during a first session and assessment. However, it can be a huge thing for a client to discuss their failings and failures with a stranger, so it can be better to do this later. Chapter 25 contains a script which focuses on the fear of failing and Appendix 25.1 includes a form which can be used to list and detail information about what the client considers to be their failures.

## The benefits approach

The benefits approach in hypnotherapy is often used with clients for smoking cessation, medical problems and pain management. In my own practice, I like to use it for a wide range of problems and hence why I have included a question about benefits in the list above. If the hypnotherapist is going to talk about failing and failures with a client, then I think it is equally important to talk about benefits; and to revisit the subject of benefits in more than one session. If benefits have already been discussed (either earlier in the assessment or in a previous session) it is important to discuss them in more depth after discussing failures and sometimes more benefits will be cited. Appendix 5.4 presents a form which can be used to record the details of each benefit.

## Using a script to identify regrets

Part III of this book contains scripts which will help to identify and acknowledge regrets which need to be worked on. However, there could be times when the hypnotherapist is already working with a client and thinks that regrets need to be identified and worked on but the client has not actually used the word "regret". The script below can be used for such situations, whereby the hypnotherapist can introduce the idea of regrets and get the client to focus on their own regrets. This can be followed by a further assessment as discussed above.

## The script: To identify regrets

Today I want us to think about regrets. Every person has regrets. Some may be very trivial – others may be more significant. I am sure there must have been times when you have regretted the choice you have made. Like being indecisive in a shop about buying an item of clothing e.g. a jumper, so you go to other shops to have a browse around. Then you decide you should have got the jumper you saw in the first shop and when you go back it has gone. Or when you cannot decide what to order in a restaurant; eventually you decide to narrow it down to two choices and then you choose one. When the meals arrive at the table, you see someone else has what you decided not to order and it looks so much better than your meal. Maybe you decide to walk home rather than waiting for the bus. When you are halfway home it starts raining heavily and by the time you get home you are soaked through. So these are all regrets but nothing really major that is going to alter the course of your life.

We can learn from the regrets we have. We know we cannot change the past but we can change how we think about it and learn from it. I think it might be useful to think about your regrets. Let your subconscious mind bring forward regrets – important regrets – significant regrets – maybe some that you have completely forgotten about. So just relax – keep breathing slowly – let things happen naturally. You do not need to force anything. Your subconscious mind will help you remember and will bring forward anything that it thinks needs some attention. Some of your regrets will have been dealt with and need no further attention. Other regrets may need attention and for you to take some action.

Just let your mind drift and drift – go right back as far as you can remember – back to when you were a baby, a toddler and then a small child. Go right back to when you were born and up to when you started school.

*(Guidance note: the hypnotherapist should then work through periods of the client's life and identify any regrets they may have had, but also acknowledge that not all regrets will need to be worked on i.e. some will not be significant or will have been dealt with already. The form in Appendix 5.2 can be used to record the regrets identified)*

Do you remember having any regrets:

In the womb?
As a baby?
As a small child?
As an older child?
In adolescence?
As a young adult – from being 18 years of age to being 21 years of age?
In your (20; 30s; 40s; 50s; 60s; 70s; 80s as appropriate)
In the last 5 years?
In the last 2 years?
In the last year?
More recently?

What do you consider to have been the major or significant regrets you have had in your lifetime?

Have you had regrets that seemed to be very significant at the time but now you consider them to be minor or insignificant?
How have these regrets affected you?
How do you feel when you regret something?
What have you learnt from thinking about these regrets?

Well done. You have worked hard to bring forward your regrets and now we know what you need to work through.

## Appendix 5.1: Questions for assessment

### *QUESTIONS FOR ASSESSMENT*

Name:                                                    Date of birth:
Address:
Telephone/mobile:
Email address:
Significant people (family/friends/colleagues):
Any professionals involved:
Reason for referral:

1.  What regrets do you have?
2.  Do these regrets stem back to:
    –   Distant past
    –   Recent past
    –   Childhood
    –   Adolescence
    –   Adulthood.
3.  How often do you think about the regrets?
4.  When do you think about the regrets?
5.  Is there any particular time you think about them? (*e.g. day; time; anniversary of an event*)
6.  Do you dwell on them? If so, for how long at any one time?
7.  Do you think regularly about any particular regret? If, so how regularly?
8.  When you reflect on your regrets what do you feel?
9.  Describe your emotions.
10. Does having these regrets affect your life now? If so, how?
11. Have these regrets affected your life in the past? If so, how?
12. Do you want to do anything in particular in regard to your regrets:
    –   Make amends
    –   Put things right
    –   Find someone
    –   Find out the truth
    –   Solve a mystery.
13. What do you think will gain from working through your regrets? Think about the benefits:
    Benefit 1:
    Benefit 2:
    Benefit 3:
    Benefit 4:
    Benefit 5:

## Appendix 5.2: Form for recording regrets identified

### *REGRETS IDENTIFIED*

Name of client:                                        Date:

**Time in life regret occurred**                **Regret: Detail/information**

1.  Any past lives identified

2.  When in the womb

3.  At birth

4.  Baby (first year of life)

5.  Toddler (up to 2 years)

6.  Young child (2 to 5 years old)

7.  Older child (6 to 12 years old)

8.  Adolescence/teenage years (13 to 17 years old)

9.  Young adult (18 to 21 years)

10. 20s

11. 30s

12. 40s

13. 50s

14. 60s

15. 70s

16. 80s

17. 90s upwards

18. Last 5 years

19. Last 2 years

20. Last year

21. More recently

22. Other

## Appendix 5.3: Form for mind mapping regrets

Name of client:                                   Date:

## Appendix 5.4: Form for recording benefits identified

### *BENEFITS IDENTIFIED*

Name of client:                                              Date:

**Benefit**                                        **Details: what will be gained**

1.

2.

3.

4.

5.

6.

7.

8.

9.

10.

# Chapter 6

# Groupwork for regrets

I have always really liked facilitating groups both in my role as a social worker and as a hypnotherapist. Groupwork is not for everyone, but if you do enjoy working in this way then it is possible to set up a group to focus on regrets. In general, groups can be set up for support purposes (e.g. a carers group; a bereavement group) or they can be set up for therapeutic purposes. When considering running a regrets group, it is important to be clear what the objectives are for such a group and then there will be other things to consider and decisions to be made e.g. regarding the lifespan of the group. One tends to think of support groups as ongoing and perhaps a long-term resource. In contrast a group set up for pregnancy and birthing will be time-limited[1].

When considering setting up a group to work on regrets there are several options the hypnotherapist might want to consider. A group which is going to deal with regrets can be run as a:

- One-off meeting for a small group of participants (I would suggest a maximum of 6) to acknowledge and identify regrets
- Time-limited group
- Ongoing group.

Running just one meeting for a group can be really effective for participants who perhaps struggle to talk about their regrets and how they are affected by having certain thoughts and feelings. Hearing other people's experiences facilitates acknowledgement that it is natural to have regrets and often can then be followed by disclosure. This type of group can be run for a half-day or a full-day session. The hypnotherapist may want to run one-off groups solely for the purpose of identification and acknowledgement of regrets (Stage 1 of the process), but it can also be a useful way of assessing people and then offering therapy in individual sessions. The hypnotherapist can develop an initial treatment plan after the group has taken place, but is more likely to undertake further assessment work before developing an in-depth treatment plan.

As mentioned above groups can be run for support or therapeutic purposes; or a combination of both. A group which is going to meet for more than one session

DOI: 10.4324/9781003468325-7

needs to have clear objectives about what it is trying to achieve (i.e. the outcomes) and within what timescale this will take place. Support groups are usually ongoing, i.e. not time-limited. It is possible to set up a time-limited group with a view to participants continuing to meet after the therapy has finished in order to offer support to each other (without the hypnotherapist).

It can happen that a hypnotherapist is working with individual clients who have regrets and thinks it may be a good idea to bring these clients together for groupwork (if they want to participate). Therefore, some groups can be created to meet a particular common need.

I want to express some thoughts about the age of participants. I have run many types of groups during my career and in particular for 21 years (until the end of 2021) I ran therapeutic support groups for adults who had been abused either in childhood and/or adulthood for an organisation I founded – Beyond Existing[2]. Initially, the groups were set up for older people and then more groups were created for anyone over the age of 18 years. What became very clear during that time was that having people of different ages in a group worked really well. In one group we had a 17-year-old girl (who was almost 18 so was allowed to join a group) and a 93-year-old woman. They developed a wonderful supportive relationship which continued years after that particular group finished.

I am raising the subject of age because people can experience different types of regrets at various stages of their lives; just like people can experience different types of losses. However, as people get older death is likely to become more prominent in their lives as relatives, friends and colleagues die. A hypnotherapist may wish to set up a group purely for people who have experienced bereavement and have regrets about what they did not say or do, which is a very common problem. Having said that, at the other end of the age scale, a bereavement group can be set up for children who have lost siblings with the same objectives in mind. Another example of groupwork is for people who have previously bullied or harassed someone, committed a crime and really regret what they did. This can be really helpful when adults regret things they did in their youth.

## Planning to set up a regrets group

Even if the hypnotherapist is experienced in running groups, they will have to put in some time thinking about why and how they want to set up a regrets group. If the hypnotherapist has no experience at all in running a group, they should discuss what they want to do in a supervision session or with someone who is experienced in groupwork; and then undertake some formal training in developing groupwork skills. I also think it is helpful to read as an introduction some of the older, well-established texts on groupwork by Tom Douglas[3], Allan Brown[4] and Mark Doel and Catherine Sawdon[5].

Appendix 6.1 includes the following questions the hypnotherapist should ask themselves when they are considering setting up a regrets group and can be used as a checklist to work through and record the decisions made:

- Why do I want to run a regrets group?
- Do I actually have the skills to run a group? Or do I need to take some specialised training?
- Who will attend the group? (consider age; gender; types of regrets being experienced; other relevant issues/circumstances/commonalities)
- How many people will be in the group? (consider minimum and maximum numbers)
- What types of regrets will be considered/worked on?
- What are the main purposes/objectives of the group? (counselling, therapy, mutual support; other objectives)
- What do I want to include in the meetings?
- What will be the content? (presentations; information/handouts; how the hypnotherapy will be delivered; methods; techniques; use of scripts)
- What will be the structure of the meetings? (e.g. how much time will be allocated for talking in the conscious state; how much time for trance work)
- Will the group be: a one-off meeting; time-limited or ongoing?
- If the group is time-limited, how many meetings will there be?
- What will be the duration of each group meeting?
- How often will the group meet?
- When will the meetings take place? (daytime/evening)
- Where will I run the group?
- What equipment might I need for groupwork?
- What shall I charge for attending the group?
- Will I take a deposit before the group starts?
- What methods of payment should I offer?
- Do I want to get feedback from group participants? If yes, how will I do this?
- Will I use a feedback/evaluation form at the end of each meeting or when the group terminates (for time-limited groups)?

## Assessment before the group starts

As stated in the previous chapter, a hypnotherapist will have their own way of assessing potential clients. Some offer an assessment by having a conversation on the telephone or online; others will do a full assessment during the first face-to-face session with a client. Before running a group, it is essential for the hypnotherapist to get as much information as possible from a potential participant. Sometimes by talking to people you get a feel of who might work well together or who might not! I suggest that it is good to have a verbal chat on the telephone initially, then to send the potential participant a questionnaire to complete (for an example questionnaire see Appendix 6.2). The hypnotherapist might feel another verbal conversation is needed with the potential participant to clarify any queries or get more detail from the information given in the questionnaire.

## Confidentiality and consent

Before attending a group meeting the hypnotherapist must discuss in full with a potential participant:

*   Confidentiality and its limits
*   Written notes/records (and where they will be stored) in order to be compliant with the *Data Protection Act 2018 and General Data Protection Regulation UK* (January 2021)
*   Audio recordings if they are going to be used and their storage (as above to be compliant).

A consent form will need to be signed. It is fine for the hypnotherapist to use their normal consent form, but some may want to design a bespoke consent form for the group. A generic consent form is included in Appendix 6.3.

## Opening exercise for a group

Once a group has come together it is important to build rapport but participants are probably going to be quite nervous initially. It is a big thing to talk about regrets, which are very personal, to a group of complete strangers. Therefore, it can be helpful to begin by talking about minor regrets to break the ice. Once trust is established the more significant regrets can be broached.

### Exercise 6.1: Thinking about regrets

**Purpose of the exercise:**

*   To introduce the subject of regrets
*   For participants to get to know something about each other
*   To focus on **minor** regrets, which are no longer significant.

**Equipment needed:** the hypnotherapist will need to have the following resources prepared in advance for this exercise:

*   Lots of plain white paper for writing on: big enough to be folded up (but not too big as to give the impression a lot needs to be written down!)
*   Pens
*   A box.

The hypnotherapist should explain the objectives of the exercise before giving each participant three pieces of paper. Everyone is asked to write down three **minor** regrets – one on each bit of paper – and preferably from three different stages of their life: childhood, adolescence and adulthood. Participants are encouraged to give some detail i.e. not just one word or two words, but not to write an essay! The hypnotherapist might want to put a limit on the number of sentences that can be written. The pieces of paper are then folded up and put in a box. The hypnotherapist shakes up the box and then asks each participant to pick out just one piece of paper and read it to themselves. The hypnotherapist should explain that if by chance a participant picks out one of their own regrets they do **not** have to disclose that to the group.

Each participant then reads out what is on the piece of paper they have picked out of the box. When everyone has read out one regret a general discussion about all the regrets is facilitated by the hypnotherapist. Participants are told they do not have to own their regrets unless they want to do so. There will be three rounds of doing this until all the regrets have been discussed. The hypnotherapist will then facilitate more discussion to ascertain how the participants are feeling. Some possible questions are:

- How do you feel after doing that exercise?
- What has it made you think about the subject of regrets in general?
- What has it made you think about your own regrets?
- What has it made you feel about your own regrets?
- Does anyone want to share one of their more significant regrets?

I think it always good to do a short relaxation session in the trance state after this exercise has been completed and then take a break. The hypnotherapist will then continue the meeting as planned.

The two exercises contained in Chapter 4 can be used in a regrets group in order to focus on:

- Emotions and introduce the idea of thoughts feelings and behaviours (Exercise 4.1)
- One specific regret and then to identify the thoughts, feelings and behaviours associated with that regret (Exercise 4.2).

## Feedback and evaluation

At the end of every group meeting it is important to have some wind-down time, so that the group participants can give some verbal feedback about how they are feeling and how they found the meeting i.e. what was useful/not useful. If the group is time-limited, the hypnotherapist may want to undertake a formal evaluation. There are various ways this can be undertaken:

- Verbally: face-to-face as a group at the end of the final meeting
- Written evaluation: completed by participants before they leave the final meeting

- Written evaluation: given out at the last meeting and to be returned by post/email
- Written evaluation: emailed after the last meeting has taken place.

For evaluations that need to be returned it can be useful to ask participants to return the form by a certain date. On occasions I have followed up participants 3, 6 or 9 months later for evaluation purposes. Again this can be done verbally or by designing a further evaluation form.

The hypnotherapist will have their own objectives for the evaluation i.e. what they want to know, but usually some feedback will be helpful about the practical things as well as the content of the sessions:

- Day/time
- Location/venue
- Original reasons/objectives for attending the group and desired outcomes: whether they were achieved
- Content of the meetings
- Methods used
- The hypnotherapist
- What was helpful/not helpful
- If anything could have been done differently
- Benefits from attending the meetings
- Any negatives.

Evaluation forms can be presented in many different formats e.g. full of questions, tick boxes for multiple choice answers or the standard:

Very satisfied [   ] Satisfied [   ] Not very satisfied [   ] Not at all satisfied [   ]

Very likely [   ] Likely [   ] Not very likely [   ] Not at all likely [   ]

Grading 1 to 10 (1 = low/not satisfied/not good); 10 = high/satisfied/good)
I do not think it is particularly helpful for an evaluation form to be just a tick box exercise. Open-ended questions need to be included as well so the participants can give some really valuable feedback (good and bad) to the hypnotherapist. The questions should be designed by the hypnotherapist to get the information/feedback they need to help and develop their practice in the future.

## Being a group facilitator and self care

None of us ever stops learning, so running a regrets group can teach the hypnotherapist many new things and can add skills to their tool box. Running a regrets group can be so rewarding, but also very demanding and challenging at times. Therefore, the hypnotherapist who runs such a group needs to take care of themselves and consider what support they might need. The hypnotherapist could consider running a group with another hypnotherapist so there are two group facilitators. This has many advantages for planning and running the group sessions; but also for debriefing purposes. Whether running a group alone or with a co-facilitator it is essential that the hypnotherapist has a proper debrief with someone after a group meeting has taken place. That someone should be a person who has the necessary knowledge about hypnotherapy, groupwork and regrets in order to support the group facilitator and to promote their wellbeing.

## The rest of the book for groupwork

The five stages of the process for working through regrets discussed in earlier chapters are relevant for and can be used in a regrets group. The group meetings can be structured to follow the stages and scripts from the rest of the book can be used or adapted if required.

## Appendix 6.1: Checklist – Key questions for the hypnotherapist before setting up a regrets group

• Why do I want to run a regrets group?

• Do I actually have the skills to run a group? Or do I need to take some specialised training?

• Who will attend the group? (consider age; gender; types of regrets being experienced; other relevant issues/circumstances/commonalities)

• How many people will be in the group? (consider minimum and maximum numbers)

• What types of regrets will be considered/worked on?

• What are the main purposes/objectives of the group? (counselling, therapy, mutual support; other objectives)

• What do I want to include in the meetings?

• What will be the content? (presentations; information/handouts; how the hypnotherapy will be delivered; methods; techniques; use of scripts)

• What will be the structure of the meetings? (e.g. how much time will be allocated for talking in the conscious state; how much time for trance work)

• Will the group be: a one-off meeting; time-limited or ongoing?

- If the group is time-limited, how many meetings will there be?

- What will be the duration of each group meeting?

- How often will the group meet?

- When will the meetings take place? (daytime/evening)

- Where will I run the group?

- What equipment might I need for groupwork?

- What shall I charge for attending the group?

- Will I take a deposit before the group starts?

- What methods of payment should I offer?

- Do I want to get feedback from group participants? If yes, how will I do this?

- Will I use a feedback/evaluation form at the end of each meeting or when the group terminates (for time-limited groups)?

## Appendix 6.2: Assessment questionnaire for a regrets group

STRICTLY CONFIDENTIAL

### ASSESSMENT QUESTIONNAIRE FOR A REGRETS GROUP

Please answer the following questions as fully as you can

Name:                                                    Date of birth:

Address:

Telephone/mobile:

Email address:

Significant people in your life (e.g. family; friends; colleagues):

Any counsellors/therapists/professionals you are currently seeing:

1.   What are your main reasons for wanting to attend a regrets group?


2.   Have you seen a hypnotherapist before? (If yes, how was that experience? Was anything particularly helpful or unhelpful?)


3.   How much do you know about hypnosis?


4.   How would you describe your general state of health?


5.   Do you have any diagnosed medical conditions? (If yes, please give details)

6. Do you ever experience any breathing difficulties e.g. asthma; hay fever? (If yes, do you use an inhaler?)

7. Have you ever had an operation? (If yes, please state when and what for)

8. Are you taking any medication? (If yes, please give details)

9. Have you ever been referred to a psychiatrist? (If yes, for what reason?)

10. Have you any fears or phobias?

11. What are your interests/hobbies?

12. How do you currently relax?

13. Is there any other information you think might be helpful to know before the group meetings start?

Form completed by:
Date:
Time:

## Appendix 6.3: Example of a standard consent form

### CONSENT TO TREATMENT, CONFIDENTIALITY AND INFORMATION SHARING

I declare that I understand and agree with the following statements:

- I shall engage in hypnosis/receive hypnotherapy treatment from (*name of hypnotherapist*).
- The limits of confidentiality have been explained to me and I have had the opportunity to discuss this and to ask any questions about things I do not understand.
- On some occasions sessions may be audio-recorded; this will not happen unless I agree.
- Everything discussed in hypnosis/hypnotherapy sessions or information given in other ways (e.g. telephone, written documents, emails, text messages) will remain confidential to (*name of hypnotherapist*) unless a concern arises about: i) a client who may harm him/herself or another person; ii) a child may be at risk of harm/abuse or iii) there are legal reasons which necessitate the sharing of information.
- Where someone is at risk of harm/abuse this information may be shared with others on a "need to know" basis (e.g. acting under the *Children Act 1989/2004*; the *Crime and Disorder Act 1998*; the *Domestic Violence, Crime and Victims Act 2004*; the *Domestic Violence, Crime and Victims (Amendment) Act 2012*).
- Written notes will be taken by (*name of hypnotherapist*) during sessions and will be stored safely in the office(s) of (*name and address of hypnotherapist*).
- Records are also kept in electronic files in the office(s) of (*name and address of hypnotherapist*).
- All records (written and electronic) will be stored safely and kept in accordance with requirements stated under the *Data Protection Act 2018* and the UK General Data Protection Regulation (1st January 2021). The retention period being up to [X] years.
- (*Name of hypnotherapist*) can contact me by:

Telephone   [   ]      Text   [   ]      E-mail   [   ]      Letter   [   ]

Name of client: ................................................................................................

Date of birth: ...................................................................................................

Address: ...........................................................................................................

Email address: ..................................................................................................

Signature: .........................................................................................................

Witnessed by: ........................................................ (*Signature of hypnotherapist*)

Date: Time:

## Notes

1 For detailed discussion about setting up such a group see Chapter 4 'Running a group' in *Hypnotherapy for Pregnancy and Birthing: Scripts for Hypnotherapists* (2022) Abingdon, Oxon: Routledge.
2 Pritchard, J. (2003) *Support Groups for Older People Who Have Been Abused: Beyond Existing.* London: Jessica Kingsley Publishers.
3 Douglas, T. (2002) *Basic Groupwork* (2nd edition). Abingdon, Oxon: Routledge.
4 Brown, Allan (1992) *Groupwork Practice* 3rd edition Abingdon, Oxon: Routledge.
5 Doel, M. and Sawdon, C. (1999) *The Essential Groupworker: Teaching and Learning Creative Groupwork.* London: Jessica Kingsley Publishers.

# Part II

# Scripts for the first session

Chapter 7

# Relaxing into your hand

## Introduction

A good way to introduce a client to trance can be to get them to focus on an object. I often bring a variety of things with me into the therapy room for this purpose. For example in autumn, I often bring in different coloured leaves. I also regularly use flowers and abstract artwork. Using objects is especially helpful when working with children to give them something to focus on. I regularly use feathers and glitter wands. The script presented below gets the client (adult or child) to focus on one of their hands in order to relax them into the trance state. It is also a useful script to teach the client self-hypnosis.

It can be helpful to use this script in conjunction with the script "Introducing the road of regrets" (see Chapter 10). Hypnotherapists work in different time slots. Some prefer to do 50-minute sessions; others like myself prefer to do longer sessions – up to one and a half hours or two hours. The amount of time available will also depend on whether the hypnotherapist has done a full assessment on the telephone or online before the first session or whether the assessment will be done face-to-face during the first half hour of the session. If the hypnotherapist offers shorter sessions, I would suggest using the script in the first session as an introduction to trance and then repeat it in the second session before working with the concept of the road of regrets. Alternatively, in a longer first session both scripts can be used together.

## The script

I want you to make yourself comfortable in that chair – really comfortable. So move about if you need to do so until you feel really comfortable. You are going to start to relax. I know you may be wondering what this is going to be like as this is something you have not done before, but there is absolutely nothing to worry about. Relaxing is a really good thing to do. It is important that everyone takes time out during the day to relax and shut out everything else that is going on. It is beneficial to take time for yourself and focus on you. Going into trance is a perfectly natural state. In order to shut things out it is helpful to focus on just one thing – to

DOI: 10.4324/9781003468325-9

look at an object – a shape – a colour maybe. Just make sure you are sitting comfortably in that chair and keep your breathing nice and slow.

I wonder if you have ever thought about how useful your hands are or do you just take them for granted. Your hands are really useful tools – they can do so many things. Today one of your hands is going to help you relax. Now I want you to choose one of your hands to concentrate on. Are you going to focus on your right hand or your left hand? OK – now hold that hand in front of you – with the back of the hand facing you. Hold it in a position which is comfortable for you – do not strain your arm. Hold your hand where you can see it clearly. You need to be able to get a really good view of your hand. Keep your breathing nice and slow as you concentrate on your hand.

Look at the back of your hand. Just take a look at the four fingers – the first finger – the index finger – the ring finger – and the little finger. Then look at your thumb. Now look at the flat bit of your hand running down into your wrist. Now take a closer look at your fingers. Follow the outline of your four fingers. Look at how they are sized differently. Now follow the outline of each finger – one at a time. The first finger – take a look around the outside of it. Start at the bottom – go up one side – over the top – and down the other side to the bottom. Now the index finger – take a look around the outside of it. Start at the bottom – go up one side – over the top – and down the other side to the bottom. Next the ring finger – take a look around the outside of it. Start at the bottom – go up one side – over the top – and down the other side to the bottom. The little finger – take a look around the outside of it. Start at the bottom – go up one side – over the top – and down the other side to the bottom. Now look at your thumb – follow the outline of your thumb. Start at the bottom – go up one side – over the top – and down the other side to the bottom.

Now look at your fingernails – one at a time. Keeping your breathing nice and slow. Look deep into the nail on the first finger – look at the shape – the colour – the different shades of dark and light within the nail. The more you look at the nail you feel as though you are being drawn in and the more relaxed you are becoming. Relaxing more and more. Then move on to look deep into the nail on the index finger – look at the shape – the colour – the different shades of dark and light within the nail. Relaxing more and more. Now move on to look deep into the nail on the ring finger – look at the shape – the colour – the different shades of dark and light within the nail. Relaxing more and more. Now move on to look deep into the nail on the little finger – look at the shape – the colour – the different shades of dark and light within the nail. Relaxing more and more. Now move on to look deep into the nail on your thumb – look at the shape – the colour – the different shades of dark and light within the nail. Relaxing more and more.

A lot of people think their knuckles are the bony, lumpy bits across the middle of their hand. You actually have a lot of knuckles – in fact you have three sets of knuckles on your fingers plus two knuckle joints on your thumb. Stretch your fingers out – now bend the tops of your fingers just below the nails. That is one set of knuckles. Look at the skin covering the knuckles. Focus on the lines running across the skin. Follow those lines. Stretch your fingers out again – now bend your fingers in the middle. That is the second set of knuckles. Look at the skin covering the knuckles. Focus on the lines running across the skin. Follow those lines. Now clench your hand – make a fist – and you will see the third set of knuckles across the middle of your hand. Look at the skin covering the knuckles. I wonder if you can see any bone showing through. Focus on the skin across your knuckles. Stretch your hand out again and look at the skin covering each finger – look at each finger – one at a time. Travel up and down each finger looking at the skin – the lines – the shapes and patterns on the fingers – one at a time. The first finger – the index finger – the ring finger and the little finger.

Now stretch out your hand and look at your thumb – bend your thumb – you will see two knuckle joints. Look at the skin covering each knuckle joint. Focus on the lines running across the skin. Stretch out your thumb. Look at the skin covering that thumb. Look for the lines – the shapes and patterns on the thumb.

Stretch out your hand again and look at the flat bit of your hand underneath the third set of knuckles. I wonder if you can see some veins standing out of your hand. Look at the skin there – see if you can see anything else on the skin – spots – marks – lines – patterns and shapes. Clench your hand – tight. Stretch it out again and then clench it tight again. Feel how soothing it is to watch your hand – stretching and clenching – stretching and clenching – stretching and clenching. Keep watching your hand – stretching and clenching – stretching and clenching – stretching and clenching.

Now turn your hand over so that you are looking at the inside of your hand. Remember to keep holding your hand in a position which is really comfortable for you – do not strain your arm. Hold your hand where you can see it clearly. You need to be able to get a really good view of the inside of your hand. I wonder if it feels different looking at the inside of your hand.

Just take a look at the four fingers – the first finger – the index finger – the ring finger – and the little finger. Then look at your thumb. Now look at the flat bit of your hand running down into your wrist. Now take a closer look. Follow the outline of your four fingers. Look at how they are sized differently – the first finger – the index finger – the ring finger – and the little finger. Now look at your thumb – following the outline of your thumb.

Do some stretching and clenching again – stretch and clench – stretch and clench – stretch and clench. Watch where your four fingers bend – they bend in three places. Stretch and clench – stretch and clench – stretch and clench. Stretch your hand out now – look at the lines running across where your fingers bend in three different places on each finger. Now concentrate on each finger – one at a time. Look at the first finger – look at the lines running across where the finger bends in three places. Look deep into those lines. Follow those lines. Take your time – no need to rush – follow those lines. Look at the index finger – look at the lines running across where the finger bends in three places. Look deep into those lines. Follow those lines. Take your time – no need to rush – follow those lines. Look at the ring finger – look at the lines running across where the finger bends in three places. Look deep into those lines. Follow those lines. Take your time – no need to rush – follow those lines. Look at the little finger – look at the lines running across where the finger bends in three places. Look deep into those lines. Follow those lines. Take your time – no need to rush – follow those lines.

Now look at your thumb – it bends in two places. Look at the lines running across where the thumb bends in two places. Look deep into those lines. Follow those lines. Take your time – no need to rush – follow those lines.

Now look into the palm of your hand. So many lines. Big lines – small lines. Long lines – short lines. Some lines cross over each other. Some lines come to an abrupt end. Look deep into the palm of your hand. Follow the lines – so many lines – so many, many lines. I am going to be quiet for a short while you follow the lines.

*(Guidance note: for an adult the hypnotherapist can be quiet up to two minutes; for any child under 16 years of age 1 minute will suffice)*

Keep looking into the palm of your hand. Look deep into the skin. You know the lines are there but I wonder what else you can see on the skin – within the skin. Look for any patterns and shapes. I am going to be quiet for a short while you look for any patterns and shapes.

*(Guidance note: as above – for an adult the hypnotherapist can be quiet up to two minutes; for any child under 16 years of age 1 minute will suffice)*

You are feeling relaxed now – your hand has helped you to relax – it is going to help you to relax even more now. You are going to relax into your hand. You are going to look at the lines again and then follow them. You can go in whichever direction you want to take. As you follow the lines you are going to relax even more and more – and your eyelids will start to feel heavy. Look deep into the palm of your hand. You are relaxing into your hand. Follow the lines – so many lines – so many, many lines.

You are feeling so relaxed now – your eyelids are feeling heavier and heavier. Your hand has helped you relax – it is going to help you to relax even more now. You are going to relax even more into your hand. You are going to look at the lines again but at the same time watch for any patterns or shapes you may see. As you look for any patterns and shapes you are going to relax even more and more – and your eyelids will start to feel heavy. Keep looking at the lines – keeping looking for any patterns and shapes – and as you are doing this your eyelids will become heavier and heavier – so very heavy. Your eyelids will become so heavy you will have to close them. Look deep into the palm of your hand. You are relaxing into your hand. Look for the lines – look for any patterns and shapes. Your eyelids are getting heavier and heavier as you are relaxing into hand. Close your eyelids when you cannot keep them open any longer. Just relax into your hand – going to deeper and deeper – deeper and deeper.

Chapter 8

# Breathing and listening to sounds

## Introduction

I developed the original version of this script when I was working with a non-visual client. He was actually fine about being non-visual and it was clear at the outset he was auditory. So I wanted to develop a script for him (and future auditory clients) using sounds and it developed from an exercise I used to do with my supervisor, Mary Sarjeant[1], at the beginning of some supervision sessions. For the purpose of this book I have adapted the script so that it can be used in an initial session. It can also be used in future sessions and will be good for any client who is predominantly auditory.

If a client is not visual they can sometimes feel like they are failing in some way during a first session. Even though a hypnotherapist will have explained about the senses and how people experience trance differently, it can sometimes take a considerable amount of time for the client to be convinced it is fine not to be visual and that they may sense things or hear things. It is vital that the hypnotherapist explains this in detail at the start of any therapeutic relationship.

In my own practice during a first session I usually talk to the client about breathing and we practise different ways of breathing in the conscious state. I then choose a method to relax them which incorporates the breathing we have been practising. I regularly refer to number, ratio and colour breathing. In my hypnotherapy book for pregnancy and birthing[2], Chapter 10 goes into detail about different types of breathing. I have reproduced the information about number and ratio breathing in Appendix 8.1 as I thought it would serve as a useful summary to read before using this script.

I have found that this particular script works really well with children; especially those who find it difficult to concentrate. Listening to sounds distracts them and can get them into trance very quickly and easily.

## The script

Close your eyes and let's do some number breathing in and out to the count of *3*. Breathe in: *1, 2, 3* – and hold

DOI: 10.4324/9781003468325-10

Breathe out: *3, 2, 1* – relax.
Breathe in: *1, 2, 3* – and hold
Breathe out: *3, 2, 1* – relax.
Good now see if you can go to *4*.
Breathe in: *1, 2, 3, 4* – and hold
Breathe out: *4, 3, 2, 1* – relax.
Breathe in: *1, 2, 3, 4* – and hold
Breathe out: *4, 3, 2, 1* – relax.

Good. Now just continue to breathe at your own pace but remember to keep breathing slowly – there is no need to rush anything. In a few moments time I am going to stop talking because I want you to listen to sounds – the sounds in the room – and any sounds you might hear outside of the room – any sounds at all. Listening to sounds can be very relaxing and it can be amazing what you might hear. As you listen your mind might drift and that is absolutely fine. Just keep relaxing. So I shall be silent now. I shall not speak for a while.

*(Guidance note: when working with an adult the hypnotherapist should remain silent for up to three/five minutes. For a child, the length of time will be dependent on age. For children under 10 years of age, I usually keep silent for up to 1 minute)*

I wonder what sounds you have been hearing – what sounds you became aware of – maybe listening to sounds made you relax – drift off somewhere. Listen again now. If you are still hearing any sounds at all I want you to let those sounds drift away. Let the sounds drift far away from you. Drift far away – far, far away. If any sounds come in during the session they will not bother you at all – they will not disturb you because you will be in a deep trance state – deeply relaxed – truly relaxed – enjoying the trance state.

## Appendix 8.1: Summary of number breathing and ratio breathing

The purpose of this appendix is to give a quick summary regarding number and ratio breathing.

### Number breathing

Number breathing involves breathing in for a certain number count and then breathing out for the same count. The main objective is to slow the breathing down and be able to control it – especially when breathing out. I usually start with a count of *3* and explain that eventually (after a week) this can be increased – firstly to *4* and then after another week to *5*.

Breathe in: *1, 2, 3* – and hold
Breathe out: *3, 2, 1* – relax.

Breathe in: *1, 2, 3, 4* – and hold
Breathe out: *4, 3, 2, 1* – relax.

Breathe in: *1, 2, 3, 4, 5* – and hold
Breathe out: *5, 4, 3, 2, 1* – relax.

### Ratio breathing

This type of breathing requires more control. It involves breathing in for a certain number count and then taking double the time to breathe out. Some clients can struggle with this at first. It is good to start with *2* and *4* and gradually increase to *3* and *6*. On occasions I have had clients that build up to *4* and *8*.

Breathe in: *1* and *2*
Breathe out: *4, 3, 2* and *1*

Breathe in: *1, 2* and *3*
Breathe out: *6, 5, 4, 3, 2* and *1*

Breathe in: *1, 2, 3* and *4*
Breathe out: *8, 7, 6, 5, 4, 3, 2* and *1*.

(From: p. 59, *Hypnotherapy for Pregnancy and Birthing*, Pritchard 2022)

## Notes

1  Mary Sarjeant, psychotherapist and counsellor, sadly passed in 2019. I would like to acknowledge that the listening to sounds exercise we used to do at the beginning of some of our supervision sessions inspired me to write the original version of this script; and as with most of my scripts they change and evolve further over time.
2  Pritchard, J. (2022) *Hypnotherapy for Pregnancy and Birthing: Scripts for Hypnotherapists*. Abingdon, Oxon: Routledge.

# Chapter 9

# Fragrant oil diffuser

## Introduction

The script in the previous chapter was designed for clients who are predominantly auditory. The script in this chapter was originally written for use with clients who are referred to as being olfactory, that is, having a strong sense of smell. It is not always evident immediately if a client has a dominant sense, so this version of the script can be used for a general introduction to trance in a first session. It can also be used in future sessions for someone who is olfactory and is already going into trance on a regular basis and practising self-hypnosis.

## The script

Just close your eyes and get ready to relax both your body and mind. We are going to do some breathing to help you relax both your body and mind. In a moment I am going to ask you to breathe in very slowly and gently while I count *1, 2,* and *3*. Then I want you to hold your breath briefly – before you breathe out very slowly and gently whilst I count *3, 2,* and *1*. Shall we give this a try? OK then – make yourself really comfortable in that chair.

Breathe in: *1, 2, 3* – and hold
Breathe out: *3, 2, 1* – relax.
And again.
Breathe in: *1, 2, 3* – and hold
Breathe out: *3, 2, 1* – relax.
Breathe in: *1, 2, 3* – and hold
Breathe out: *3, 2, 1* – relax.

Just keep breathing very slowly and gently, whilst I start to ask you to imagine certain things. If you can see what I suggest that is good, but if cannot see anything do not concern yourself, because you will sense what is in front and around you – and you may even smell something. Any noises you may hear will just drift into the background. Just let everything happen naturally – there is no need to force

DOI: 10.4324/9781003468325-11

anything. You are going to become completely relaxed. You will not have a care in the world.

Just keep breathing very slowly and gently – that's right. Now I want to imagine that in front of you there is a fragrant oil diffuser. I do not know whether it will be on a windowsill – on a mantelpiece or on a shelf. Wherever it is – it is directly in front of you. Imagine the glass bottle – look at the shape of it – look for the narrow neck of it. The glass bottle has ten reeds standing tall within it. The glass bottle is filled with oil – relaxing fragrant oil. Look into the glass bottle – look at the oil. I wonder what colour it is. The oil is very smooth so it can be absorbed easily by the reeds. Just like you can absorb relaxation into your body and mind. Keep looking at the oil – smooth and relaxing. I wonder if you can smell anything.

Look at the ten reeds again standing tall in the bottle. Maybe some of them are leaning at an angle – resting on the sides of the neck of the bottle. Maybe some of them are standing upright in the middle of the neck of the bottle. Look at the reeds – notice their colour – what they are made of – maybe you can imagine what it would feel like to touch them. The reeds are absorbing the relaxing fragrant oil and the reeds are giving out a wonderful smell. Just imagine the reeds absorbing this wonderful relaxing fragrant oil. The reeds become softer as the oil is absorbed slowly and gently – they work better when they feel relaxed. As you imagine the reeds absorbing the oil, feel your body relaxing – becoming softer. As you imagine the reeds absorbing the oil, you feel your mind relaxing. You are relaxing more and more.

Look at the ten reeds again. I am going to count down from *10* down to *1*. Each time you hear me say a number you will look at a different reed and imagine absorbing the relaxing oil into your body and mind. Ready now – look at the ten reeds.

*10*: Look at one of the reeds in the glass bottle. Take a deep breath in and then breathe out – relax.

*9*: Look at another reed and relax even more.

*8.* Now look at another reed and imagine the oil being absorbed by this reed. The reed is strong as it has a job to do, but at the same it is soft and relaxed – working well – diffusing the fragrance from the relaxing oil.

*7*: As you look at a different reed, feel the relaxation moving upwards from your toes and feet – into your ankles – then into the lower half of your legs – up towards your knees and into your thighs.

*6*: Look at another reed as the relaxation is moving up and over the trunk of your body. Your stomach and chest are relaxing inside your body and outside of your body. Keep looking at a different reed whenever you hear me say another number.

*5*: The relaxation is moving into your fingers, thumbs and hands – into your wrists – then into the lower half of your arms – up towards your elbows and into your upper arms.

4:    Feel your body absorbing the relaxation as it moves up the back of you – over your buttocks – up from the bottom of your spine – to the very top of your spine.

3:    Relaxing more and more. Feel the relaxation moving into your shoulders – your neck – your throat – over your face – up the back of your head. Only two more reeds left.

2:    Take a deep breath. Breath in the relaxation – through your nose – into the inside of your head. Round and round it goes. Relaxing your mind.

1:    The last reed. Your mind is relaxing more and more now – relaxing more and more – becoming completely relaxed – not a care in the world. Take another deep breath in and then breath out – relax.

0:    Now your whole body and your mind are completely relaxed.

# Part III

# Identifying and acknowledging regrets

Chapter 10

# Road of regrets

## Introduction

I think clients find it useful to have a concept to work with or to use a metaphor through the therapeutic process when working with a treatment plan (i.e. to return to it during each session) in order to help them work towards their goals. I shall discuss this further below, but I want to explain that my practice has developed in this way because of how I started my social work career. In the early days of my career, I was working with terminally ill children in a children's hospital. I found Elizabeth Kubler-Ross' works[1] on death and dying really helpful and they grounded me. Kubler-Ross' five stages of grief have always been fundamental to my practice and have given me a clear structure when working with terminally ill children or adults; or when helping someone with bereavement and the grieving process:

1.  Denial
2.  Anger
3.  Bargaining
4.  Depression
5.  Acceptance.

I have also found the works of Colin Murray-Parkes[2] equally helpful and have regularly used and referred to his model of grief which has four stages:

1.  Shock and numbness
2.  Yearning and searching
3.  Disorganisation and despair
4.  Reorganisation and recovery.

Over the years, when working as both a social worker and hypnotherapist I have developed specific terms or metaphors to help clients. When helping a client through the grieving process I use the concept of the *journey of grief*[3]. It is helpful to work with the concept of a journey, which may have many roadworks, obstacles,

DOI: 10.4324/9781003468325-13

diversions and rerouting along the way. The idea is to work towards the final destination of acceptance. Similarly, when working with regrets, I have developed the concept of the *road of regrets* because everyone has regrets through their lifetime. Some regrets will be very minor; and will be given some immediate thought or only remembered in the short term. Others may be more significant and some can have a massive detrimental effect on the individual, which can be ongoing in the long term. It is important to acknowledge that regrets are a normal part of life; because no-one is perfect and no-one gets everything right. We all make mistakes and hopefully most of the time we learn from them.

By introducing the concept of the road of regrets, it suggests to the client that it is OK to have regrets, i.e. it is part of life. The road is one which has to be travelled along at the client's pace and in their own time. This is a very different message to what people are often told, i.e. life is too short to have regrets. The expectation being that one should "move on" or "upwards and onwards"; and not dwell on the past. With these clichés being spoken fairly regularly, it is no wonder that regrets are often not faced and dealt with in therapy. By introducing the road of regrets early on in the therapeutic process (even during the first session after a proper assessment has been undertaken), the client is given permission to have regrets and to feel regretful; and then they will be helped to work through them while following a treatment plan.

The road to be walked along will include:

- Identifying and acknowledging regrets (Stage 1)
- Working through regrets by looking back at the past and considering what happened; and identifying the associated emotions (Stage 2)
- Taking action(s) to deal with any unresolved issues (Stage 3)
- Releasing the regrets and emotions (Stage 4)
- Planning for the future (Stage 5).

Two scripts are included below, which can either be delivered together in one session or in separate sessions. Script 1 introduces the road of regrets and can be used in a first or second session to introduce the concept of the road of regrets. Some clients may already be very clear about what they regret and therefore may not have to do much work on identifying what they need to work on. It can still be valuable to use the script as an introduction with the purpose of emphasising it is normal to have regrets. The concept of the road can then be returned to in future sessions. Script 2 prepares the client for travelling along the road of regrets; and helps the client decide how they will travel along their road i.e. their own mode of transportation.

## Script 1: Introducing the road of regrets

I want you to consider how we all walk millions of steps and thousands of miles throughout our lifetimes. Think about how many steps you have walked today already. Where have you been today – what have you been doing before you came here? Think about how many more steps you might walk during the rest of the day. Think about how many steps you walked yesterday – the day before that – and the day before that. What about last week – how many steps did you walk? And last month – did you walk more or less than the previous month? And last year – how many steps did you walk? Are you counting? Are you adding up the steps? How many years have you lived? How many steps have you walked? How many steps will you walk in the future? You may not know the exact number but what you do know is you have walked a lot of steps in your life so far – since you started walking as a baby – as a toddler – as a young child – as an adolescent – and as an adult. You have walked lots and lots and lots of steps. It can be quite exhausting thinking about the number of steps you have walked, but you have walked and you have kept going. Taking more and more steps. You may have tripped – stumbled – fallen over – but you have got back up and carried on. Taking more and more steps.

Many things will happen to you while you are living your life. You will experience many different things. You will say and do many different things. Other people will say and do many different things to you. There will be times when things will not happen as you would like. There will be times when you are not happy with the way you have reacted in a situation or the way you have responded to a person. Ultimately, you will have some regrets. Regrets are a normal part of life. You will develop regrets as you experience life; there will be such a mixture of regrets. Some regrets will be of no consequence, other regrets will have a considerable and memorable impact on you.

You are here now because you want to work on your regrets – you want to work through them. To do this I want you to imagine your own road of regrets. The road you must travel. See a road in front of you now. This road contains all the regrets you have ever had. Some you may be seeing very clearly in your mind and may think about on a regular basis in the conscious state. Others may be deeply embedded within you – deeply embedded within your subconscious mind. It is important for your wellbeing to understand these regrets and to work through them. You can do this – and you will do this on the road of regrets. You will travel your own way and at your own pace along the road of regrets. This is a very private road – it is not open to the public. It is your own road of regrets.

For now though just think about this road of regrets. Look into the distance – see how long or short the road is. Look down and see what the road is made of. Look to the right and then to the left. I wonder what you are seeing. Take a deep breath – prepare yourself to travel along the road of regrets. You can travel any way you want to do so – you can walk – run – drive – fly – use any mode of transport you like. Remember you will travel along the road of regrets at your own pace – slow – quick – you can rest at any time – and you can also change direction if you need to do so. You know you need to travel along the road of regrets. You acknowledge that you need to do this. You know it will be worthwhile to focus on the regrets – identify them – and then to work through them. Take another really deep breath

– and when you are ready to start – step onto the road – your own road of regrets you need to travel along. You are ready to identify and face your regrets.

*(Guidance note: the hypnotherapist has the choice to carry on in this session using the road to identify regrets to be worked on in future sessions OR other scripts in Part III can be used for identification)*

## Script 2: Preparing for travel

We know that everyone is an individual and each person will handle things in their own way. The subconscious mind will know the best way to help and it will be there for you when you travel along the road of regrets. It is up to you to decide how you want to travel along the road regrets. You can choose your mode of transport – the speed you want to travel – you are going to do whatever is best for you. It is perfectly OK to change your mind too. The way you think and the way you feel about things may change along the way, so that may change the way you travel and it may also change your speed. It is also fine to take a rest whenever you want – or to change direction if you need to do so.

You know you have got a lot of work to do. Like training for a marathon, you need to work hard and put in a lot of effort. That is why I want you to think about the road of regrets you are going to travel along and what things you might have to face. There may be things you expect to encounter and have to deal with, but there may also be unexpected incidents, events, things you had forgotten.

So now it is time to start travelling along the road of regrets. How would you like to start travelling today?

*(Guidance note: clients often come up with very imaginative ways to travel. However, the hypnotherapist can use the following prompts and then may use additional scripts from other parts of the book)*

Would you like to:

Walk (*or stroll; skip; jump; run*)
Cycle
Drive
Ride (*e.g. a horse; in a carriage*)
Fly?

So you have chosen your way to travel. Take some deep breaths and start to prepare yourself to find the regrets along the road. Take some more deep breaths to prepare yourself to face your regrets. Take some more deep breaths to prepare yourself to work through your regrets. You are ready and you are prepared. You can and you will travel along the road of regrets. Now start travelling and tell me what you see.

## Notes

1 Kubler-Ross, E. and Kessler, D. (2014) *On Grief and Grieving: Finding the Meaning of Grief Through the Five Stages of Loss.* London: Simon and Schuster Inc. Elizabeth Kubler-Ross' original work *On Death and Dying* was written back in 1969 and there have been many anniversary editions produced since then. It is worth reading a version. She wrote many other books too; all of which will enrich a hypnotherapist's knowledge and understanding of death and dying, but also regarding grief and grieving.
2 See Parkes, C.M. and Prigerson, H.G. (2010) *Bereavement: Studies of Grief in Adult Life* 4th Edition. London: Penguin; Parkes, C.M. and Markus, A. (1998) *Coping with Loss.* London: BMJ Books.
3 Chapter 6 'Journey of grief' in *Dealing with Different Types of Losses Using Hypnotherapy Scripts* by Pritchard, J. (2022) Abingdon, Oxon: Routledge.

Chapter 11

# Riding the regrets

## Introduction

Travelling along the road of regrets is not usually a smooth ride; the client is likely to come across a lot of bumps along the way – in this script the bumps are waves. When riding a jet-ski out to sea, the client faces the waves when they are both rough and calm. The script can be used soon after introducing the concept of the road of regrets, but it can be used again whenever the client struggles with travelling on their own road of regrets. It is an effective script, which can be used in any session (and as often as needed) as the treatment plan is worked through.

## The script

I understand that when you have regrets and especially when you are working through them, it can feel like everything is topsy-turvy. Travelling along the road of regrets can be turbulent. I want you to remember that you have a terrific imagination and there are ways that you can ride the regrets – ride over them – to find calmness and tranquillity. Remember you are strong and you are resilient.

I want you to imagine that you are on a beach – a beautiful beach with white sand. Look out towards the sea – see how blue it is. You can see some people swimming in the sea. There are a few people on the beach – some lying on towels – others on loungers. Some children are making sandcastles. As you look towards the sea again you notice that there are some jet-skis at the water's edge. Walk down towards the jet-skis. As you get nearer a person comes towards you and gestures for you to choose a jet-ski. Have a good look at the jet-skis – they are all different colours. Choose the one you would like to ride on the sea. Then push the jet-ski into the sea and climb on it. Make yourself comfortable on the seat and put your feet in the footwell. Become familiar with the different parts of the jet-ski – the handlebars – and different levers on the handlebars for the throttle – to go forward – to reverse – to brake. Sometimes you may need to travel backwards as well as forwards. At other times you may need to stop suddenly when something unexpected happens. Take hold of the handlebars and feel confident that you can drive the jet-ski and ride the waves. You are in control. You can drive the jet-ski and ride the waves.

DOI: 10.4324/9781003468325-14

Look out to sea – watch the waves – coming in and out – rising up and down. Coming in and out – rising up and down. Take some deep breaths and switch on the ignition. The jet-ski is ready to go and so are you. You are in control and ready to ride the waves. Start moving forward – start travelling over the water – over the waves. Keep your eyes on the waves. Riding over them – up and down – up and down. You are enjoying the ride – enjoying the movement – enjoying being in control. Watch how the waves move – you see that they can become bigger – more forceful. Then they can subside – grow smaller. It is a bit like regrets – on some days they feel more powerful as though they are taking you over – dominating your life. On other days they feel smaller – they do not intrude so much. It is hard to predict how the waves will be – it is hard to predict how the regrets will make you feel. Remember – you are in control. You know that you can ride the waves on the jet-ski just like you can ride the regrets – whatever they throw at you. You just need to relax and go with the waves – up and down – up and down.

Keep driving forward on the jet-ski. Watch the waves. Up and down – up and down. I wonder how your stomach is feeling – a bit queasy perhaps. Just like when you think about your regrets. I wonder if there have been times when you have felt nauseous or even been physically sick (*or insert anything else the client has previously described*). Just imagine feeling nauseous and being sick (*or insert anything else the client has previously described*) now as you ride the waves. Keep tight hold of the handlebars – ride the waves – ride the waves – up and down – up and down. Keep going until the nausea and sickness *(or insert anything else the client has previously described)* passes. Well done. You rode the waves well.

Sometimes a regret can come into your mind very suddenly and unexpectedly. It makes you feel off kilter – knocks you sideways. Just like when a big wave comes out of nowhere. Look at the sea again – look at the waves – you are riding the waves – up and down – just as you have been doing on the journey so far. Then suddenly out of nowhere you a see a huge wave coming straight at you – you need to think quickly – you need to act quickly. Use the brake lever on the handlebars to stop. Then start again – change the direction of the jet-ski. Hold on tight to the handlebars and steer away or reverse away from the wave – that's right. You manoeuvred the jet-ski – instinctively you knew what to do. Well done. You changed direction when you needed to do so. You knew what to do. You were in complete control.

Now keep riding the waves. You are ready to face anything that is thrown at you. You know you can ride your regrets. Tell me what it feels like when you are riding the waves – thinking about your regrets.

What is going through your mind?
What do you see in front of you?
What is coming at you?

Now the waves are smaller. The sea is calm. It is time to return the jet-ski to the water's edge at the beach. Before you do that – have one last ride – enjoy the peaceful sea – enjoy being in control – you know you can face anything – you know you can ride the waves.

Chapter 12

# Tea bags and coffee granules

## Introduction

I would say that in the majority of cases, hypnotherapists find themselves working with regrets when the client has brought up the subject of regrets either in the initial assessment or when in the trance state during a session when a treatment plan is already in place. However, sometimes a client may say they are feeling regretful but they find it difficult to explain what they regret exactly. The two short scripts in this chapter can be used to identify regrets by working with tea bags or coffee granules. It is important to ascertain whether a client does like drinking tea or coffee (and their preference if they have one) before choosing which script to use. It is also useful to remember that some people do not like or drink either beverage.

In Appendix 12.1 there is a very simple form, which the hypnotherapist can use to record the regrets which are identified. The form can be used with the other scripts in Part III of the book; but it can also be useful for recording when other regrets are identified during other stages of the process or when using scripts in other parts of the book.

## Script 1: Tea bags

You are feeling thirsty and would like to make a cup of tea. So imagine that you are in a kitchen – any kitchen – and start looking around for where the tea bags are stored. I wonder where you will find them. Maybe they are in a box in a cupboard – or in a tea caddy – or some sort of other storage container. Have a good look around and tell me when you have found the tea bags. Where were they? Now find a table and chair where you can sit down and take the tea bags with you. Look at the tea bags in the (*box, caddy or whatever type of container the client said*). Look at all the tea bags you see in front of you. Look at the shapes of the bags. Then look at the paper which contains the tea leaves. I wonder what patterns you can see on the paper. While you are looking at the tea bags feel yourself relaxing more and more – going deeper and deeper – let your subconscious mind relax – relaxing more and more. These tea bags contain many different tea leaves. Keep looking for patterns you see on the outside of the tea bags.

DOI: 10.4324/9781003468325-15

You have mentioned having regrets. Sometimes it is hard to know exactly what you regret, but your subconscious mind knows. Your subconscious mind knows everything about you. Your subconscious mind will help you to know what you regret and how you can deal with, work through and release your regrets. As you are starting to think about regrets choose one tea bag from the (*box, caddy or whatever type of container the client said*). Hold that tea bag in one of your hands. Look at it closely – focus again on the patterns you see on the paper which contains the tea leaves. Think about your regrets. Go back to your childhood – adolescence – adulthood. As you are thinking about your regrets open up the tea bag. Look at the tea leaves lying within the bag. Look deep into the tea bag. Now pick out a tea leaf and put it on the table. What is that regret?

*(Guidance note: the hypnotherapist should then encourage the client to talk about the regret)*

Tell me more about that regret.
What do you regret exactly?
How do you feel now as you are talking about that regret?

*(Guidance note: when the client has finished talking about the regret the hypnotherapist needs to find out if there are any more regrets)*

Look at the tea bag again – and the tea leaves within it. Do you see any other regrets?

*(Guidance note: if the answer is yes, then another tea leaf is taken out of the tea bag. This continues until all the regrets have been identified)*

Well done. You have identified the regrets you have. It is good to bring things out into the open. In future sessions we shall consider the effects the regrets have had on you and how they have affected your life. How are you feeling right now?

You have done a lot of work today bringing things out into the open. I think it is time for you to have a cup of tea and relax. Why don't you tidy up the tea leaves and the tea bag you have opened up and get rid of them? Now put the kettle on – find a cup – and a spoon. Find a fresh tea bag and put it in the cup. Listen to the kettle starting to boil. The water is being prepared so that you can enjoy a lovely cup of tea. Feel the anticipation – knowing your thirst will be quenched. Just like you know you will be working through your regrets in future sessions. Feel the anticipation and some excitement. Sometimes when you drink you may experience a bitter taste – and it may come as a shock. Sometimes the drink will taste smooth and soothing – and you will experience a sense of satisfaction. The kettle has boiled now – the water is ready – pour the water onto the tea bag and wait for the tea to brew. Now take some time to relax – enjoy your cup of tea.

## Script 2: Coffee granules

You are feeling thirsty and would like to make a cup of coffee. So imagine that you are in a kitchen – any kitchen – and start looking around for a jar of coffee. I wonder where you will find it. Have a good look around and tell me when you have found it. Where was it? Now find a table and chair where you can sit down and take the jar with you. Hold the jar in your hand and look at the glass – the label on the jar – and the granules inside. Look deep into the granules – look at their colour – the shape of each granule. I wonder if the jar feels heavy in your hand.

You have mentioned having regrets. Sometimes it is hard to know exactly what you regret, but your subconscious mind knows. Your subconscious mind knows everything about you. Your subconscious mind will help you to know what you regret and how you can deal with, work on and release your regrets. As you are starting to think about your regrets open the lid of the jar. Look into the jar. Look at the granules again – look at their colour – the shape of each granule.

Think about your regrets. Go back to your childhood – adolescence – adulthood. As you are thinking about your regrets pick out a granule from the jar and put it on the table. Look at the granule. What is that regret?

*(Guidance note: the hypnotherapist should then encourage the client to talk about the regret)*

Tell me more about that regret.
What do you regret exactly?
How do you feel now as you are talking about that regret?

*(Guidance note: when the client has finished talking about the regret the hypno-therapist needs to find out if there are more regrets)*

Look into the jar again – and the granules within it. Do you have any other regrets?

*(Guidance note: if the answer is yes, then another granule is taken out of the jar. This continues until all the regrets have been identified)*

Well done you have identified the regrets you have. It is good to bring things out into the open. In future sessions we shall consider the effects the regrets have had on you and how they have affected your life. How are you feeling right now?

You have done a lot of work today bringing things out into the open. I think it is time for you to have a cup of coffee and relax. Throw away the granules you picked out of jar. Now put the kettle on – find a mug – and a spoon. Spoon some coffee granules into the mug. Listen to the kettle starting to boil. The water is being pre-pared so that you can enjoy a lovely mug of coffee. Feel the anticipation – knowing your thirst will be quenched. Just like you know you will be working through your regrets in future sessions. Feel the anticipation and some excitement. Sometimes when you drink you may experience a bitter taste – and it may come as a shock. Sometimes the drink will taste smooth and soothing – and you will experience a sense of satisfaction. The kettle has boiled now – the water is ready – pour the water onto the waiting coffee granules Now take some time to relax – enjoy your mug of coffee.

## Appendix 12.1: Form for recording regrets

### *REGRETS*

Name of client:                                      Date:

**Type of regret**                                   **Details**

1.

2.

3.

4.

5.

6.

7.

8.

9.

10.

# Chapter 13

# Hanging out the washing

## Introduction

This is another script to help a client identify what regrets they actually have. In my own practice, I have come across clients who say they feel regret or regretful but they find it very hard in the conscious state to know exactly why they feel like this i.e. what has caused the feeling. Sometimes this is due to the subconscious mind protecting the client because what has actually happened is too painful to face. However, the fact that the client has come for therapy is a good indicator that the time is right to work on this feeling of regret and identify what has caused it.

This script enables the client to identify regrets using a washing line. It is a good script to use in an early session to lay the foundations for the more intensive work in future sessions. It is worth noting that on occasions the client will immediately start to do some work on a regret whilst hanging out the washing. So although the hypnotherapist's main objective in using the script is to identify the regrets and then plan for future sessions, it may be some of the work can be started immediately because the client suddenly knows what they need to do.

## The script

It is springtime. Spring is always such a lovely time of year. The weather gets better – it can be warmer because the sun shines for longer. It can be a time for new beginnings and a time for hope. It is always good to have a spring clean at the beginning of this season. Have a bit of a sort out – sort out any rubbish in the house you do not need anymore – and then have a good clean. When it gets warmer it is also nice to be able to hang out the washing so it smells lovely and fresh after it has dried in the warm rays of the bright sunshine.

Today you are going to start sorting things out – sorting out what is going on in your mind. Your subconscious mind suppresses some things to protect you and it will bring things forward when it is the right time to do so. You have been talking about feeling regretful but have been finding it hard to express what the regret or regrets actually are. So it might be a good time to have your own spring clean – sort things out – throw away anything you do not need anymore.

DOI: 10.4324/9781003468325-16

I want you to imagine that you are in a house – a house will come forward into your mind. Now have a good look round. I want you to find where the washing machine is – maybe in the kitchen or perhaps in a utility room. At the same time keep your eyes open for a laundry basket and some pegs. Tell me when you have found the washing machine. Good. Now look through the glass on the door. You will see there is a whole heap of wet washing in the drum – the cycle has finished. Open the door and take out all the items. Just hold them in your hands and see how heavy they feel. The washed items are very tangled up. It is very easy for things to get mixed up – knotted up – tangled. Now put the tangled items in a heap in the laundry basket.

Go outside into the garden taking the laundry basket with you – and you will see a long washing line. It is time to start untangling the washing. Start doing that now – untangle the washing. At the same time, I want you to experience those feelings of regret again as you untangle the washing. Keep untangling. It can be hard untangling those items of washing that have got mixed up – knotted up – tangled. Keep untangling. Experience those feelings of regret now. Keep untangling the washing and as you do so place each washed item in a pile in the laundry basket. As you are untangling the washing you start to understand what you regret exactly. It becomes clear in your mind what the regret is. You may have just one regret or there may be several – sometimes they are interlinked or joined up – tangled like the washing. It will benefit you to think about any regrets you may have and identify what you actually regret.

There is no rush. Keep untangling and looking at the items of washing in the laundry basket – all clean and fresh. Keep untangling. When you feel ready you will pick up an item and feel the material. Look at the item – look deep into the item. You will see a regret.

*(Guidance note: the hypnotherapist should encourage the client to name the regret and then talk about it. Some questions and prompts are given below. Not all of them will be relevant to each regret)*

Tell me what the regret is.
Give it a name.
Talk to me about the regret.
What happened?
What do you regret?
How do feel as you look at the regret?
How do you feel as you are holding the regret?

Now get some pegs from the laundry basket and hang (*regret*) on the line. Stand back and look at (*regret*).

What are you thinking?
Is there anything you want to do about this regret?

Keep looking at the regret on the washing line for a while longer. Have you got any other thoughts or feelings about this regret?

OK so now look again at the pile of washing in the laundry basket. See if there are any more regrets in the laundry basket.

*(Guidance note: repeat the process with another item if the client does see another regret in the laundry basket)*

Well done you have hung out all the washing and you have identified your regrets. For now, just stand back and look at the washing on the line. It starts to blow. The sun is shining so it will not take long for the washing to dry. Once it is dry you will have the ironing to do which is another task I know you can do well. Ironing can be so satisfying – smoothing things out – removing the creases and bumps – making things look just as they should be.

Chapter 14

# Hunt the thimbles

## Introduction

This is another script which can be used to identify regrets by playing the game "hunt the thimbles". It is an ideal script for working with children, but works equally well with adults. It is impossible to predict or know how many thimbles will be found, so on occasions when a lot of thimbles (regrets) have been hidden it may be necessary to continue the hunt in the next session.

## The script

I am sure you know that there are lots of different games people play which involve finding things. For example, on Easter Sunday children go outside and hunt for Easter eggs. Human beings hide themselves when playing hide and seek. I wonder if you have ever played hunt the thimble. When you think of a thimble I wonder if you think of someone sewing and wearing a thimble to protect their thumb or finger from being pricked. Thimbles can make it easier to push a needle through thick material. Thimbles can be made from all sorts of strong materials – rubber – leather – china – glass. A thimble is a very useful thing to have because not only can it protect you, it is a useful place to hide things. Your subconscious mind is a bit like a thimble – it does its best to protect you. Just like a thimble protects someone who is sewing from getting pricked – hurt.

Everyone has regrets – some are of no consequence at all – others could be very important and impact on your life greatly. Whether a regret is big or small, it is important to acknowledge it and deal with it so it has no further impact. There are times when it is necessary to hunt for the regrets – bring them out into the open – and then get rid of them. To do this, you are going to play a new version of hunt the thimble. I want you to imagine that all your regrets are in thimbles, which have been hidden in your house – and maybe other places too. I have no idea but you will know. So just imagine you are in your house. You know the thimbles have been well hidden – they are out of sight. You need to search everywhere to find them. Before you start searching, find a big black bag so you can throw away the thimbles once you have looked at the regret. Get a really big, strong black bag.

DOI: 10.4324/9781003468325-17

Remember that some regrets will not be significant and you can throw the thimble straight into the black bag. Other regrets will be significant. They will have affected you and impacted on your life. They will have affected the way you think – the way you feel – and the way you behave.

Imagine you are in your house.
Where are you exactly in your house?
Where would you like to start hunting for the thimbles?

OK – off you go. You need to go into every room and search really hard – under furniture – on shelves – in drawers – in cupboards – under cushions – under rugs – in between clothing – in shoes – boots – trainers. There are so many place where the thimbles could be hidden. Keep searching and tell me when you find a thimble.

What does the thimble look like?
What is the thimble made of?
Shake the thimble and let the regret fall into the palm of your hand.
What is the regret?
What do you see?
Is the regret significant in some way? If yes, tell me more about that.
Has the regret affected you in the past? If so, how has it affected you?
Is this regret affecting your life now? If so, in what way?

*(Guidance note: if the regret is not significant then the client can throw away the thimble and continue the hunt for other thimbles. If the regret is significant, the hypnotherapist should encourage the client to talk about the regret and gain information to plan for the work that needs to be undertaken in future sessions)*

What do you regret exactly?
Tell me more about this regret.
What do you need to do about this regret?

OK so you have done well finding that thimble and talking about that regret. Throw that thimble into the big, strong black bag. It is no longer serves a purpose. It protected the regret for as long as it needed to do so – it did a good job – but now it is time for you to work on that regret. So keep hunting for other thimbles. Whereabouts in the house are you now?

*(Guidance note: the hunt will continue and as the client finds thimbles the process will be repeated. The hunt will continue until no more thimbles are found. It is also necessary to check that the client does not need to go to any other place in order to hunt for more thimbles. If thimbles are not found in the house it may be necessary for the client to hunt outside e.g. in the garden, back yard, shed, garage etc)*

Is there anywhere else you need to go to hunt for thimbles?

Well that was a good game but it was also a very purposeful game. You now know what regrets have been significant for you and now you can go forward and work through those regrets. Now the game is over, make sure you get rid of that big, black bag. Do that now – throw away all the thimbles.

# Part IV

# Working through emotions

# Chapter 15

# Pathway through the woods

## Introduction

This script can be used to regress the client, who will take a walk into some woods and choose a pathway, which will lead them back in time to help gain understanding and clarity about an event or situation which has caused a regret. Ideally the script should be used after the regrets have been identified in a previous session (Stage 1 of the process along the road of regrets); and will facilitate the next stage of working through the regrets (Stage 2). The script can be used as many times as necessary to work on different regrets. Towards the end of the script there is a section which involves having a picnic. This can be used to continue working through the regrets to ascertain whether the client needs to take any specific action (Stage 3) before releasing the regret (Stage 4); or it can be used to work solely on the future (Stage 5).

## The script

When you think about going for a walk you probably think about walking forward. You walked into this room coming forwards. I wonder if you can remember the last time you walked backwards – or sideways – or in another way – perhaps diagonally. Think about how many times you have walked differently – not forwards.

Think now about the possibility of going to walk in some woods. Some quiet woods where there are so many beautiful trees. All different shapes and sizes. Some will be very old – with thick trunks and gnarled bark – and lots of branches. Others may be younger – thinner – and have fewer branches. Look at the trees – there is so much to see. Look at the trunks – the branches – the leaves. So many different shapes and patterns to look at – be drawn into. As you are looking at the trees you became aware that you are standing on a pathway. You feel drawn to move forward. So do that – walk forward along the pathway. Look around you – at all the beauty in the woods. So many things to see and explore. I wonder if you are hearing any noises – or maybe smelling anything in the woods. Keep walking forward along the pathway.

DOI: 10.4324/9781003468325-19

As you continue walking in the woods, you see different pathways opening up in front of you. I wonder how many pathways you can see. As you approach the different pathways you know that some will take you forwards and some will take you backwards. Some might take you on a short cut. Others might take you a long way round. Sometimes it is necessary to go backwards – backward in time – to see what you left behind or to remember what happened – and understand why something happened. It can be useful to know why you said or did something – or why you reacted in a particular way to a person in a certain situation – or how you felt like you did then and how you feel like you do now. Going backwards – backward in time – can help you understand – give you some clarity – and then you can go forwards.

Keep walking – looking at the different pathways. Now stop walking. Tell me how many pathways there are. Now it is time to choose a pathway that will take you back in time. Back to the time when something happened that has since caused you to feel regretful. Just stand where you are and look at the pathways. Take your time – no need to rush. Tell me when you have chosen the pathway that will take you back in time.

OK – turn around so your back is facing that pathway. It is now time to walk backwards. It may feel strange at first – you may feel a bit awkward because you do not walk backwards very often. Start slowly – one step at a time – start slowly – walking backwards along the pathway you have chosen. Slowly – take another step. Good. Keep walking backwards.

As you continue to walk backwards you are going back in time. Back to the time when something happened – an event, incident or situation that has since caused you to have regrets. Keep walking backwards – going back in time – back in time to where you need to be – to gain understanding – to gain clarity. Keep going back in time until you know you need to stop – you will know you have arrived. Tell me when you stop walking backwards.

Now on the count of 3 I want you to turn around – *1, 2,* and *3.*
Tell me where you are.

*(Guidance note: the hypnotherapist should then work with the client to relive the event/situation and release the feelings associated with it. The hypnotherapist will create their own questions as the situation unfolds but some general questions follow below)*

What are you seeing or sensing?
Where are you?
Is anyone else there?
What is happening?
What do you do?
What do you say?
What happens next?
How are you feeling?

Now turn around and find another pathway. Walk forwards until you see the same event/situation in front of you. When you see it – stop. Now think about what you would do differently. Let the situation play out as you would want it to do.

*(Guidance note: the hypnotherapist will be led by the client but will facilitate the reframing of the event/situation)*

What have you learnt from coming down this pathway?
How do feel about the regret now?

*(Guidance note: there may be other regrets that need to be worked on. The hypnotherapist may choose to continue in the same session to find another pathway to regress the client or the woods can be returned to in a future session. When all the regrets have been dealt with and the client is ready to consider the future the ending below should be used)*

## Ending: The picnic basket

Well done. You have done a lot of walking backwards which can be exhausting, but congratulations on the work you have done. Facing the past can be hard but also very worthwhile to get some understanding and clarity. So now it is time to relax and think about walking forwards into the future. Now that you have dealt with the past it is good to think about what you want to do now and in the future – what you want to achieve – maybe set some goals. So choose a fresh pathway – walk forwards – and somewhere along the pathway you will find a picnic basket. So start walking forwards – feeling relaxed – confident –optimistic – hopeful – look for the picnic basket. Tell me when you find it.

Good. Now keep going along the pathway until you find an opening where you can sit and make yourself comfortable. It is time to have a picnic. Tell me when you have found a good spot. Sit down and make yourself comfortable. Feeling relaxed – confident – optimistic – and hopeful. Look at the picnic basket. Describe it to me. This picnic basket holds all sorts of things. It has everything you might like to eat and drink when on a picnic but it also holds things for the future. So on the count of *3* – open the picnic basket and take out the food and drink – *1, 2,* and *3.* Sort out the food and drink – and take some refreshment for yourself – you have been working hard – you need to build up your strength. Enjoy the food – enjoy the drink. What do you like best?

Now that you are feeling refreshed, it is time to take another look in the picnic basket. The picnic basket contains things for your future. Things you want to do – things you want to achieve. Sometimes it is necessary to take some positive action before you can move forward into the future and achieve what you want. I just wonder if there is anything you need to do – anything you need to resolve – in relation to the regret(s) you have been working through. Your basket may contain things to help you and will also show you things for your future.

*(Guidance note: the hypnotherapist may want to insert specific suggestions here e.g. finding a person; have a conversation with someone; make amends in some way etc. Alternatively, the objective can be to set goals for the future)*

Have a good look into the picnic basket – put your hand right into it. What do you find?

*(Guidance note: discussion will follow about what the client brings out of the picnic basket)*

Is there anything else in the picnic basket?

*(Guidance note: the client will keep looking into the basket until everything has been brought out)*

So now you know what you want to do and what you want to achieve in the future.

# Chapter 16

# The square to the past

## Introduction

This is another script that uses regression to take the client back in time to work on the regrets and release the emotions associated with the regret(s). This is done by visiting a square and entering a house. The client may regress to a time in their current life, but the hypnotherapist should not be surprised if they regress to a past life. Regrets can be carried from one or more past lives into the current life when issues have not been resolved. In order to heal, the emotions attached to those regrets and which have been carried through the lives, have to be released.

The script can be used more than once i.e. in following sessions. Sometimes the client will go to the same house on the square, but the hypnotherapist should be prepared for the possibility that the client will go into a different house. I have included some simple questions/prompts for hypnotherapists who have not undertaken specific training on past life regression or reincarnation therapy.

## The script

I want you to imagine that you are sitting in a beautiful old square, which is located in the heart of a modern city but you would never know that. It is surrounded by big houses that were built many, many years ago. The square may seem more like a rectangle in shape rather than a square, but it has always been referred to as the square. There are four sides to the square – north – east – south – and west. A road goes around the four sides of the square in front of the houses. Then in the middle is the area where you are sitting now. It is a like a huge garden. Look around the area where you are sitting – there are railings surrounding this area where people come to have some peace and quiet by themselves or to meet with someone. People sit – talk – eat – drink – read – relax. Children play and enjoy themselves – it is important to have fun. There are grassed areas – paths – flowerbeds – trees – and benches.

Now look at the houses – they are surrounding all four sides of the square – north – east – south – and west. Each house looks different. This is because they were all built at different times. Look at the houses on each side of the square – north – east – south – and west. Each house has many stories to tell as so many

DOI: 10.4324/9781003468325-20

individuals and families have lived here. Many people have worked on building the houses or lived in them. There are so many stories to be told. Look at what the houses are made of – some will have bricks – others will be built of stone. Look at the front doors. Look at the windows. They are all so very different. Some have steps up to the front door. Others have a flat path leading directly to the front door. Some have small gardens in front of the house – others have paved areas.

Now as you are sitting so comfortably there in the square, I want you to think about the regrets you have. I shall be silent for a minute or so while you think about your regrets.

*(Guidance note: the hypnotherapist should remain quiet for between one and two minutes)*

It is now time to go back in time. Your subconscious mind is going to work with us to identify what has caused you to have the regrets – what happened – what was significant. Your subconscious mind will take you back – back in time – to a place in time you need to be. Take another look at the houses around the four sides of the square – north – east – south – and west. Keep thinking about your regrets as you look at the houses. Look again at the houses around the four sides of the square – north – east – south – and west. You will feel drawn to a particular house. You will know which house you need to go into. When you are ready stand up and walk towards the house that you are drawn to. As you walk from the square you will be walking back in time. Walk out of the area surrounded by railings and walk towards the house you are drawn to. Going back – back in time – to a place in time you need to be. Tell me when you are standing in front of the house.

Tell me what the house looks like.
Does the house has a number or a name?
What is the front door made of?
What colour is it?
Can you see anything else on the front door?

Now you are going to go back in time. You are ready to look at your regrets – to see what happened. On the count of *3* you will open the front door of the house – *1, 2,* and *3* – open the door and in you go. Back and back in time. Close the door behind you. Back and back in time. Take a deep, calming breath in and then breathe out very slowly. Take another deep, calming breath in and then breathe out very slowly. Look around you.

*(Guidance note: the hypnotherapist should be prepared for the fact that the client may go back to a time in their current life or they may go back to a past life. The following questions/prompts can be used if required)*

Where are you?
What is happening?
What are you doing?
Is anyone else there with you?
What happens next?
Is there any conversation?
Tell me what is happening now.
How are you feeling?

*If the client has regressed to a past life:*

Who are you?
Do you know your name?
Are you: male/female/boy/girl/man/woman?
What are you wearing?
What have you got on your feet?
Do you know how old you are?
Do you know what year it is?
Do you know where you are? *(e.g. country/town/city)*
Go to a significant event.

*(Guidance note: the hypnotherapist will encourage the client to relive the event. This may need to be done several times. It is vital for the client to re-experience the emotions they felt at the time and then release them. It is helpful to ask the client to grade the emotional pain between 1 and 10. 1 being little pain and 10 being very strong/extreme pain. The event should be relived as many times as necessary until the pain is 0)*

It is time to come out of the house and go back to the square. Find the door of the house. Now open the door – go back outside – and shut the door behind you. Now go and relax in the square. Take some time for yourself. Just relax in the square.

Chapter 17

# Russian dolls

## Introduction

The main aim of this script is to help the client to look at different versions of themselves during their lifetime and to consider the regrets they have had and may still have. This is done by imagining a set of Russian (or nesting) dolls. This script works well with both adults and children. However, some younger clients may never have seen a set of Russian dolls. I have a toy/resource box, which contains all sorts of things, that I carry with me when working with children/young people. A hypnotherapist might want to have a set of Russian dolls in their resource box.

The script can be used to identify regrets initially and then can be used again for more in-depth work in other sessions. Appendix 17.1 includes a form which the hypnotherapist might like to use to note the regrets that are identified; and Appendix 17.2 includes a form to plan future work. The dolls are used to take the client back through their lifetime, i.e. a regression technique is being used. A doll can take the client back to a significant event related to the regrets. It is impossible to know how many dolls may be revealed and consequently the script may need to be used in more than one session.

## The script

I wonder if you have ever seen a set of Russian dolls. Some people refer to them as nesting dolls. They are dolls that live inside of each other. There is one big doll with little dolls of varying sizes inside. They are usually made of wood and beautifully painted on the outside. I want you to imagine that you are holding a Russian doll in the palm of one of your hands. Now hold it in both hands. Feel the smoothness of the wood. Now look at the doll. Look at the head – the face. See how all the facial features are drawn in such detail. Look at the eyebrows – the eyes – the nose – the mouth – the jaw line. You feel there is something familiar about this doll. Now look at how the doll is dressed. Look at the clothes – the colours that you can see. I wonder what the doll has on its feet.

Look at the doll again. It may seem very familiar. It is a bit like looking into a mirror. You notice now that there is what looks like a line running around the

DOI: 10.4324/9781003468325-21

middle of the doll. Touch it with your fingers – let your fingers feel the line going round the whole of the middle of the doll. You realise that the doll can come apart. Place both hands on the doll and turn it – the doll unscrews in the middle. The doll comes apart and you find another doll inside. This doll is slightly smaller. Take this doll out of the bottom of the big doll and place it to one side. Put the two halves of the big doll next to it.

Now look at the smaller doll. Look at the head – the face. See how all the facial features are drawn in such detail. Look at the eyebrows – the eyes – the nose – the mouth – the jaw line. You feel there is something familiar about this doll. Now look at how the doll is dressed. Look at the clothes – the colours that you can see. I wonder what the doll has on its feet. Look at the doll again. It does seem very familiar. It is a bit like looking into a mirror.

These two dolls will remind you of you. There is the big doll – the you as you are now. Inside there are other dolls – other versions of you – you as you have been previously. You as you have evolved through your lifetime. Unscrewing the dolls can reveal what has happened to you. The dolls can tell you what happened exactly – what you thought – what you felt – how you behaved and why you have regrets now. It can be helpful to look back in order to remember and to understand. The dolls are going to help you to do this. I do not know how many dolls will be within the big doll but you will know how many you need to reveal and talk to.

So pick up the first doll – hold it in your hands. Feel how smooth the outside of the doll is as you hold it in your hands. Tell me about the present you. What regrets are you holding in your hands?

*(Guidance note: the hypnotherapist should then work with the client to identify the regrets they have now. When they have been identified and talked about the regrets in depth, the hypnotherapist will go to the next doll and repeat the process. The client will talk about their regrets whilst holding the doll in their hand. The form in Appendix 17.1 can be used to take notes about the regrets)*

So now you have finished talking about that doll – place it to one side. Now pick up the second doll – hold it in your hands. Feel how smooth the outside of the doll is as you hold it in your hands. Think about this previous version of you. Tell me about that you.

*(Guidance note: the hypnotherapist facilitates discussion about the regrets which link to another time in the client's life)*

How are old are you?
What happened then?
What regrets are you holding in your hands?

OK I wonder if there are more dolls to find. Find the line going round the middle of the doll you are holding – and unscrew it – see if there is another doll inside. If there is another doll – take it out – and put the two parts of the doll you are holding to one side for now and pick up the smaller doll. Feel how smooth the outside of the doll is as you hold it in your hands. Think about a previous version of you. Tell me about that you. What regrets are you holding in your hands?

*(Guidance note: when all the dolls have been revealed continue as follows)*

You have found *(insert number of dolls revealed)* dolls. You have identified times in your life when you have had regrets and you know what regrets you are still carrying now. It is important to understand why a person feels like they do. It is important to know that you may not be able to change what has happened in the past but you can change how you think about it and how you feel about it. It is important to remember that you have a future – the time to take action regarding the regrets and then to plan for your future.

What would you like to do?

*(Guidance note: whilst still in trance the hypnotherapist can identify what needs to be worked on in future sessions. The form in Appendix 17.2 can be used for recording the work to be done)*

## Appendix 17.1: Form for regrets identified using the Russian dolls

*REGRETS IDENTIFIED*

Name of client:                                          Date of session:

**DOLL**                   **TIME IN CLIENT'S LIFE**                   **REGRETS**

First doll

Second doll

Doll 3

Doll 4

Doll 5

Doll 6

Doll 7

Doll 8

Doll 9

Doll 10

## Appendix 17.2: Form for identifying work to be done

### *WORK TO BE DONE*

Name of client:                              Date of session:

**REGRET**                                **WORK TO BE DONE**

1.

2.

3.

4.

5.

6.

7.

8.

9.

10.

# Chapter 18

# Under the microscope

## Introduction

With the aid of a microscope the client explores their thoughts, feelings and behaviours in relation to their regrets. It enables the hypnotherapist to gain more information and then if necessary amend or develop a more detailed treatment plan. As the client travels along their road of regrets it may be necessary to amend or develop the treatment plan which is currently in place.

## The script

There may be times when we do not want to look at ourselves. There could be many reasons for this. Maybe we are afraid of what we might see. Whatever the reason there are times when we do need to look at ourselves and learn from what we see. We need to look at the outside and we need to look at the inside too.

When we have regrets it can be helpful to take a look at ourselves in order to understand how we think – how we feel – and how we behave. It is necessary to look back in time to what happened and also to look at how we are now. It may be difficult facing this but it will be beneficial. Some understanding and clarity will be gained. Although we need to take a deep look into thoughts, feelings and behaviours it can be done from a distance if required.

Imagine that you are in a science laboratory. There will be benches and stools in there and lots of scientific equipment. I want you to take a look around and see what there is. As you wander around look out for a microscope. Keep looking and tell me when you have found the microscope. Good. The microscope is going to help you see things more clearly because it has a very powerful lens. It magnifies things – makes them appear bigger so you can get a really good view. Now place the microscope on one of the benches and make yourself comfortable on a stool. Take some deep, slow breaths – in and out – in and out. That's right – deep and slow. In a moment you are going to look at your regrets through the microscope. You will feel perfectly calm and safe doing this – yes you will – calm and safe.

It is a good thing to look at your regrets and think about how they affect your thoughts and feelings – and how your thoughts and feelings can affect your

DOI: 10.4324/9781003468325-22

behaviour. You need to gain some understanding and clarity about why you have thought about your regrets the way you have – why you have experienced the feelings you have and why you have behaved as you have done. It will be beneficial to understand why your regrets have affected you and continue to do so.

So once again just take some deep, slow breaths – in and out – in and out. That's right – deep and slow. Start thinking about the regrets you have been carrying with you. Think about each individual regret. What happened or did not happen. Think about what you regret exactly. When you are ready you are going to take a look into the microscope and the regrets you have will be clearly visible. Are you ready to take a look now? Take a deep breath and look into the microscope.

Look down – see the regrets you have been carrying with you. If you need to see more clearly turn the focusing knob on the side of the microscope so that you get a really clear view. See the regrets you have been carrying with you very clearly. The microscope is going to help you understand why you think, feel and behave as you do about these regrets.

How many regrets do you see?
Now separate them out under the microscope. You need to consider and understand each regret – one at a time.
Which regret do you see first?

*(Guidance note: at this point the hypnotherapist needs to explore the regret. A number of questions are listed below to help the hypnotherapist. Not all of them will be relevant to the regret which is being looked at under the microscope. The objective is for the hypnotherapist to gain as much information as possible from the client about what they regret exactly and explore their thoughts, feelings and behaviours)*

What is the regret?
Tell me about the regret.
What do you regret exactly?
What happened *(or did not happen)*?
When did this happen *(or not happen)*?
What were you thinking at the time this happened?
What do you think about it now?
How often do you think about this regret?
Over time, what feelings have you experienced in relation to this regret?
What feelings do you have about it now?
How long have you felt this way?
Can you explain the reasons for feeling this way?
Is there a reason you have not been able to let this feeling *(or feelings)* go?
What caused you to feel this way?
How did you behave in that situation?
What did you do/say in that situation?
What did you not do/say in that situation?

Has having this regret changed your behaviour in anyway? If yes, tell me more about that.
When you are thinking about this regret, how do you behave?
When you are thinking about this regret, what do you do?

Well done in acknowledging how you think about that regret – how you feel about that regret – and how you have been behaving because of carrying this regret with you. Now it is time to ask yourself whether you need to take any action so that the regret is dealt with and the emotions attached to it can be released.

*(Guidance note: many types of regret could be presented by the client, so the hypnotherapist's suggestions need to be adapted to suit the regret. Below are just some suggestions)*

Some people need to have a conversation with someone – to ask questions or to explain something. Others may feel they should follow an ambition – chase/rectify a missed opportunity. What might you need to do?

*(Guidance note: once this regret has been dealt with if other regrets have been seen under the microscope the process will be repeated. The session should then be finished with some ego boosting)*

Chapter 19

# Walking in the rain

## Introduction

Regrets can come and go into one's thoughts. It can be quite random how often this happens. They can come suddenly and unexpectedly maybe with no obvious reason or trigger, but cause emotional distress or pain. Some regrets can also come into the mind more frequently as time goes on depending on their significance. Some may eventually be at the forefront of one's thoughts for a large part of the day and sometimes night (causing disturbed sleep). By walking through the rain, the client will see their regrets in the raindrops. Various feelings will be experienced – heaviness, stickiness, being glued together or stuck. The purpose of the script is to embed the idea that the client will weather the storm i.e. they will deal with the regrets and go forward.

## The script

Close your eyes and imagine that you are somewhere outside. It is a very dull day. The sky is full of grey clouds. It looks like it is going to rain. Start walking forward – take some deep breaths in and out – focus on your breathing. Keep walking forward. You feel something cold drop on your nose. Then it happens again. More cold drops fall onto your forehead – your cheeks – and your chin. It has started raining. It feels like a light shower. You look up and see the raindrops falling from the clouds. Stand still for a moment and watch the raindrops falling. Look at the shape of each one. Look through each one. They fall gently and lightly. Keep watching.

As you are watching the raindrops, think about the regrets you have. Regrets can make you experience many different emotions and it can help to talk about the regrets and how they make you feel. So continue your walk in the rain and at the same time keep looking at the raindrops. Watch the raindrops carefully. In some of the raindrops you will see a regret. The regrets you need to deal with will fall in some of the raindrops. Watch the raindrops carefully. Tell me when you see a regret.

DOI: 10.4324/9781003468325-23

*(Guidance note: the hypnotherapist then encourages the client to talk about the regrets and the following questions can be used to explore the feelings the client is experiencing in relation to that regret)*

Tell me about that regret.

What do you regret exactly?

How does it make you feel when you look at this regret?

Can you see other regrets in any of the raindrops which are still falling?

*(Guidance note: sometimes the client may only see one regret. However, if the client does see more regrets in the raindrops, the hypnotherapist should repeat the questions in order to learn more about the regrets and the feelings associated with each one)*

The rain is starting to fall more heavily now. You need to keep walking – you need to get out of the rain. The rain is getting heavier and heavier. The raindrops are falling quickly. The raindrops fall onto the top of your head – face – hands – clothes – shoes. Your clothes are becoming wet through – saturated – you feel the dampness and wet coming through to your skin. Your clothes are sticking to you like glue – it feels like your clothes are stuck to you. Your clothes feel heavy. You feel sticky – glued together – stuck.

The rain is getting heavier and heavier now. The wind is getting up. It is making it hard to walk forward. Then suddenly there is a flash of light across the dark sky. Lightening. It is so unexpected. You do not know where it will strike next. Lightening is like a sharp pain – it strikes – makes its presence known – and then it is gone. You are waiting for it to occur again. Then there is a big rumbling sound which ends in a bang. Thunder. Crash. Such a loud noise. Your ears are ringing. You feel taken aback – off balance. Somehow everything feels different around you.

All this started from a few raindrops falling lightly. Raindrops full of regrets. Raindrops can grow in strength and effect. Raindrops can develop into a thunderstorm. Just like a regret can start off niggling at you – you think about it a bit – then you think about it more. You experience different feelings. You carry the regret around – thinking about it more and more. It sticks to you like glue. You feel stuck with it. It is painful. It is heavy. You never know when the regret is going to come into your mind again – you are waiting for it to happen – for it to make a sudden appearance – quick as lightening. Then there it is again – in your thoughts – bang and crash.

You need to face any regret and work through it. Do not hide away or try to find shelter. You can deal with the regret and move forward. Just like you can walk through a light rain shower – or a heavy rain shower – and face lightening and a thunderstorm. You can and you will walk through it all.

Now keep walking through the thunderstorm. You can do this. You are resilient. Keep walking – keep going. Walk through the storm. The rain starts to feel lighter. The sky starts to look less dark. Keep walking – keep going. You can and you will reach dryness. Keep walking – keep going. The raindrops are getting fewer and fewer. The rain is becoming lighter and lighter. The rain is stopping. The rain has now stopped completely. The sky is brightening. The clouds are disappearing. You see a bit of blue in the sky. Keep walking – keep going. Then suddenly the sun comes out. You feel the warmth on your face. You have got through the rain – you have got through the thunderstorm – and now you have found the sunshine. Just like the way you will work through your regrets and move forward into your future.

# Chapter 20

# The donkey with a heavy load

## Introduction

This script is for clients who say their regrets feel like a heavy burden. So often I have clients say when describing how their regrets make them feel:

- I feel bogged down
- They are dragging me down
- I can't shake them loose.

The donkey in the script is made to work in awful conditions and carries a heavy load. By watching the donkey on its journey, the client will be focused on its strength, determination, endurance until the donkey reaches its destination and sheds it load; so it no longer feels heaviness, tiredness or pain.

In the script I have referred to the donkey as "he". The hypnotherapist should substitute "he" in the script with the client's gender pronoun so that the two match.

## The script

A donkey may seem quite small compared to a racehorse or a shire horse. You may think of a donkey as being small and quite cute. Some people say a donkey has a sad face. Bring a donkey into your mind now. How does it look to you?

Now let your mind travel to a very hot country – a country where donkeys are made to work very hard all through the day. It is a very, very hot day. Feel the sun beating down – the heat is surrounding you – enveloping you. Feel the heat all around you – above you – on every side of you – even below you as it seems like the heat is coming up through the ground. Your head is throbbing. Your skin is perspiring. You can feel the sweat running down your neck – down your back – and down your front – down your arms into your hands – and down your legs onto your feet. Your clothes are sticking to you. You only have very thin clothes on but the heat is making you feel sticky and so uncomfortable. How is a donkey going to feel in this heat with a thick hair coat covering its body?

DOI: 10.4324/9781003468325-24

A donkey is standing in front of you – standing very still. Look at his thick hair coat. Be very aware of the heat surrounding both of you. Look at the donkey again. You see he is carrying many things. Sacks, bags and boxes are tied across the donkey's back and are hanging down on either side of him. The donkey is carrying so many things it is hard to actually see his body. You are aware of his very thin, bony four legs. Look at some of the things the donkey is carrying – heavy slabs of stone – rocks – pebbles – soil. What else can you see? You wonder how the donkey is managing to stand up with all the things he is carrying – on his back – down both sides. The donkey's head is hanging low. The donkey is feeling heavy – overloaded – burdened – immobile.

There is a loud shout. The donkey perks up his ears. There is another loud shout. The donkey lifts his head – he looks forward. You can see the expression on the donkey's face change. He looks determined. His head lifts higher. Then suddenly he takes a step forward. He wobbles a bit. He takes another step forward. He wobbles a bit again. The sacks, bags and boxes sway on the donkey's back and down his sides. He takes another step forward – he is steadier now. He takes another step and then another. He is more certain – more confident. He is moving slowly but steadily forward. Watch the donkey. As he continues to go forward he starts to move more quickly. His steps forward become steadier – he appears to be more certain – more confident. He keeps going forward. His head is held high and he looks forward.

It is really hard to understand how the donkey can carry all those objects and keep going forward in the incredible heat. He is having to work in such awful conditions – he is overloaded – he is not allowed to rest – he is not given any refreshments. His body feels as though it is being dragged down – down towards the ground. His body is aching. There is no respite from the pain. Everything is so heavy – so very, very heavy.

The donkey may look small but he is strong – so very strong and so very determined. He is determined to carry the heavy load to its destination. So he keeps going, knowing that the time will come when the heavy load will be taken off him. Everything will have to be offloaded. So the donkey keeps going – going forward with his heavy load. Determined that he will reach the destination – deliver the heavy load – and get rid of the heaviness – the tiredness – and the pain. Watch the donkey on his journey – being aware of the heat – the heaviness – the tiredness – and the pain.

The donkey continues. He is determined to get the job done. He is determined to shed the heavy load and be free of the heaviness – the tiredness – and the pain. So he keeps going – on and on and on. Carrying a heavy load can have consequences – an aching back – cuts and bruises – sore hooves. The donkey keeps going. He has nearly reached his destination now – the place where the heavy load has to be delivered – offloaded. The donkey slows down as he nears the final destination. He knows he will feel relief when the sacks, bags and boxes are taken off him. He is thinking about the time when he will be free of all the objects that have been a burden to him. Things that have had to be carried a long way or for a long time need to be shed eventually. Some things cannot be carried forever.

The donkey has stopped. Some people come to take the sacks, bags and boxes from the donkey. The donkey drops his head. He is tired, but as each sack – each bag – each box is taken from him he feels lighter. He lifts his head up – he shakes his legs – one by one. He is feeling relieved that the heavy load has been taken from him.

A person will have different loads to carry through life – some will be light – some will be very heavy. Sometimes it is necessary to carry a load for a reason – there is a purpose – you learn from the experience. But you cannot carry a heavy load forever – you cannot let it drag you down. You need to shed it – offload it. You know that don't you?

# Chapter 21

# Feeling trapped

## Introduction

The feeling of being trapped is an issue which is presented in the therapy room on a fairly regular basis. It is a feeling which can be experienced when dealing with all sorts of problems but typically when working with claustrophobia or agoraphobia. I have also worked with it when someone is lacking confidence and feels that they cannot make progress in their life because of that. Similarly, it can be a feeling which is evident when someone is dealing with regrets. The focus on regrets can become overwhelming – even to the point of becoming obsessional. The regrets totally dominate the client's life so that they do feel trapped and as though there is no way out.

In the script a prison cell is used to experience the feeling of being trapped. The prisoner is taught how to use their imagination to distract him/herself (escape) and to stop intrusive thoughts. The prisoner then breaks free from the cell and experiences a sense of freedom.

## The script

You have explained to me that you often feel trapped and you cannot get away from that feeling. I know this will be uncomfortable but I want you to think of the last time you actually felt like this – the feeling of being trapped. Let your mind drift back to when you felt like this – think about where you were – what you were doing – what you were thinking – what it was like to feel that way – of being trapped. I know it will feel uncomfortable but I want you to stay with the feeling – the feeling of being trapped – experience it again. Just drift back to that situation – go back and experience that feeling of being trapped again. Let your mind drift back to when you felt trapped – think about where you were – what you were doing – what you were thinking – what it was like to feel that way – of being trapped. Stay with that feeling – experience it again. Describe to me what it is like to feel trapped.

*(Guidance note: the hypnotherapist should allow time for discussion)*

DOI: 10.4324/9781003468325-25

Now I want you to imagine a prison – a large prison that has many prison cells within it. See the prison in front of you. You may see some cars driving up to the prison. There may be people walking around or queuing up to get into the prison to visit someone. Now imagine being inside the prison. You are locked in one of the prison cells. Look around you. The cell is very small. There is only a little window which has bars on the outside – letting in a small amount of light. There is a huge door which is locked. There is a bed, toilet and washbasin. What else can you see in the prison cell?

Sit or lie down on the bed. Feel what it is like to be locked in this prison cell. There is little light in the cell which makes it difficult to see things clearly. You may hear noises – from outside the prison walls. You may hear noises from inside the prison walls. The noises become louder – louder and louder – from outside the prison walls and from inside the prison walls. The noises make it difficult to concentrate. You feel trapped because you cannot see a way out – you cannot control the noises – you have no control – you feel powerless – because you are trapped in the prison cell. What else are you feeling right now?

*(Guidance note: the hypnotherapist should explore the feelings of the client and encourage in-depth discussion about these feelings)*

There is always an end to everything. Being incarcerated in this prison cell will come to an end. You can escape – you can escape in your mind. You have the power to stop thoughts coming into your mind. You have the power to change the way you feel. You have the power to go anywhere you want to go in your imagination. You can leave the feeling of being trapped behind you. You need to believe that you have the power to change things – to escape from the prison cell and experience freedom.

So think about the regrets you have – then think about those thoughts that regularly come into your head. Those thoughts have been holding you as a prisoner in your own mind. It is time to stop those thoughts. Hold your arm out in front of you – and put up your hand – with the palm facing away from you and say "Stop". The thoughts will stop immediately. Now think about those thoughts again. Hold your arm out in front of you – put up your hand – with the palm facing away from you and say "Stop". The thoughts will stop immediately. Do that again. Bring forward those thoughts that regularly come into your head when you are thinking about your regrets. Now stop those thoughts. Hold your arm out in front of you – put up your hand – with the palm facing away from you and say "Stop". The thoughts stop immediately. They have gone. You have taken control. Those thoughts are no longer trapped in your mind.

Now it is time to unlock the door to freedom. Freedom and a future where you can live your life just as you want to do without feeling trapped (*and insert any other feeling the client has talked about*). You can do whatever you want and you can achieve anything you really want to do. You will be free to do new things – have new experiences – explore new opportunities. Look at the prison cell door.

Look at the colour – what it is made of. See the peep hole in the centre of it. See where the lock is located on the door. Now feel under the bed and you will find the key to the door. When you have found the key, hold it in your hand. Hold the key tight in your hand. The key has the power to unlock the door – the key has the power to get you out of this prison cell. As you are holding the key very tight think about the things you want to do in the future when you are no longer feeling trapped in this prison cell. Tell me about what you are going to do.

*(Guidance note: the hypnotherapist should allow time for discussion)*

Now it is time to leave the prison cell. For one last time focus on that feeling of being trapped (*and insert any other feeling the client may have described earlier*). You are going to release that feeling of being trapped and experience complete freedom. On the count of 3 you will get off the bed and walk towards the door. Ready – *1, 2,* and *3* – get off the bed now and walk towards the door. Put the key in the keyhole. Just wait while you take some deep breaths. Breathe in – and breathe out. Prepare to escape. Breathe in – and breathe out. You are ready to be free. One more time, breathe in – and breathe out. Now turn the key and on the count of *3* you will open the door and escape to freedom. Ready – *1, 2,* and *3* – open the door and walk forward. You are no longer trapped. You are totally free. Free to think – free to feel. You are free to do whatever you want. You are free to go wherever you want. Nothing is going to hold you back.

Walk along the prison corridor. Find the exit from the prison. Leave the prison. You are now outside. You are no longer trapped. You are totally free. Free to think – free to feel. You are free to do whatever you want. You are free to go wherever you want. Nothing is going to hold you back. You are free to choose how you want to live your life.

How will you live your life?

# Chapter 22

# Stuck, frozen and numb

## Introduction

In the previous chapter the feeling of being trapped was considered in the script, whereas in this chapter the word "stuck" is used because it another word that is often used by clients. The concept of being stuck is so common for clients who are working on regrets and I am often told "I cannot move on", i.e. they feel immobilised. Clients also regularly talk about feeling "frozen" or "numb". Script 1 focuses on being stuck and feeling frozen. Script 2 considers the benefits of numbness to prevent experiencing pain in the short term and ends with experiencing new sensations.

## Script 1: Stuck in the snow

You are driving a car along a road – it is just a normal day – you are going on a route you know so well. You are living your life as you normally do. As you are driving along you suddenly notice that the sky is becoming darker. You think this is a bit odd as it is the middle of the day. You keep on driving. Then you notice some snowflakes dropping onto the windscreen. The sky gets even darker as more snowflakes start to fall. You turn on the windscreen wipers so you can see clearly through the windscreen. Watching the snow distracts you a little from driving. The snowflakes start to fall more quickly so you need to make the windscreen wipers go faster. You have a sinking feeling in your stomach wondering if you will be able to carry on driving if the snow continues to fall.

You keep driving but your journey does not feel the same. Everything around you is changing. The snow continues to fall – faster and faster. You can see the snow on the road ahead. The car suddenly slips out of control and your stomach turns. Then you get back on track again. You keep driving but you slow down a bit. The snow is still falling. The road ahead is completely covered in snow – it is like a white blanket. You start to feel panicky. The snow is getting thicker and thicker on the road – hindering your journey. You do not feel in control.

The snow keeps falling – it is getting thicker and thicker on the road. You start to feel sick. You slow down even more. The car is struggling to get through the

DOI: 10.4324/9781003468325-26

snow. The wheels keep turning but the car keeps getting stuck. You keep trying to move forward. You are stopping and starting trying to make the car go forward. The wheels keep spinning round and round but the car goes nowhere. Then suddenly the car will not move at all. The car is stuck. You are stuck. You do not know what to do. There are no other cars on the road – nobody is around. There is no signal on your phone. You are stuck. You are alone. You do not know what to do.

Having regrets can make you feel stuck. It is like you cannot move forward – you are immobile. You cannot live your life as you had been doing before you had any regrets. You feel stuck – going nowhere in your life – but that is only temporary. You will find a way to become unstuck.

You wait. You stay stuck. It is not a good feeling. Time passes. You start to feel cold – very cold. You wait. You stay stuck. It is not a good feeling. Time passes. You feel frozen now – it is so very cold. Your feet and hands feel numb. It feels like you have been stuck for such a long time. You feel you cannot move – you feel that you are immobile. You wait. You stay stuck. It is not a good feeling. Time passes. You decide you have to do something. You cannot stay stuck. You cannot stay frozen. You cannot stay immobile. You suddenly remember that you have a shovel in the boot of the car. You get out of the car and get the shovel. You start to dig the snow out from around the car. You dig the snow away from the front of the car and start to make piles of snow on the side of the road. You make two lanes going in front of the car so it will be able to move forward.

You keep digging – keep moving forward. Making two clear lanes. You are moving. You are mobile. You feel you are getting somewhere now – you are progressing. You feel less stuck. You are warming up. You are not frozen anymore. You keep digging – keep moving forward. Then suddenly in the distance you see a house. You see lights on in the house. Someone will be able to help you. You keep digging along the road – making two lanes. You are almost at the house. You keep digging along the road – making two lanes. Then you reach the house. You walk back to the car and get in. You start the engine and drive towards the house where someone will be able to help you. You are moving. You are warm – you can feel your hands and feet. You are mobile. You have dug yourself out of the snow and you are on the road again.

## Script 2: Being at the dentist

I want you to imagine you are lying down in a dentist's chair. You know you are going to have some treatment which will necessitate you having to have an injection in order to numb the pain. I wonder how you are feeling as you are thinking about this. You are aware of the dentist in the room – making preparations – reading your notes on the computer. The dental nurse is there too – lining up instruments – making sure there is water in the cup so you can rinse your mouth out whenever you need to do so. She hands you a tissue to hold. I wonder how you are feeling about having the injection – having the treatment.

Sometimes it is necessary to experience a little prick in the gum, which can feel uncomfortable, but it will help to avoid you experiencing pain. Numbness can help to avoid feeling pain. So take some deep breaths – you know you can relax by slowing your breathing down. The dentist is ready now. You can see the syringe out of the corner of your eye. You open your mouth – you see the syringe coming closer and closer. The syringe is in your mouth – you are waiting to feel the prick in your gum – there it is – you feel the liquid going into your gum. Then the syringe is taken out of your mouth.

Now focus on your gum. It is becoming numb. Just a little bit at first and then the numbness spreads. Along your gum – spreading – along it goes. Your gum is becoming number and number – number and number. You feel like you have no control over your gum or that side of your mouth. It is for your own benefit – yet it still does not feel good not to be in control. That something is taking over – spreading. Having regrets can make you feel numb. It is like they take over – take over your life – you feel numb about everything else – you have no feeling. No feeling at all. But that will not last – it is only temporary.

The dentist gets to work now. Drilling your tooth – going deeper and deeper – drilling some more. Your gum and mouth are numb – you do not feel a thing. Sometimes there is a benefit to feeling numb. Numbness can protect you. The dentist continues to drill – removing the decay – drilling some more – and then finally fills the hole. At the last treatment is finished.

You take some water from the cup and swill out your mouth. You spit all the bits and debris into the little sink. Your gum and mouth are still numb so it is not easy drinking from the cup. You take another sip and swill again. Spitting out all the bits and debris from your mouth. Your gum and mouth are still numb so it is not easy drinking from the cup, but you continue. The dental nurse fills up the cup with fresh water. This begins to feel good. Your mouth feels clean and fresh. You take some more water. Then you are done. You thank the dentist and dental nurse and then you are ready to leave the surgery.

Imagine now you have reached home and you are sitting comfortably. Your eyes are closed. Focus your attention on your mouth – on the gum that was numbed. It starts to feel different somehow. You feel some sensation in the gum. It is becoming less numb. Wait for a while – then focus again. Focus your attention on your mouth – on the gum that was numbed. You feel the numbness is easing more and more. You feel that you are gaining some control back – control over your mouth. You are feeling your gum – you are feeling that side of your mouth. Be aware the numbness is going – feel your gum and mouth feeling like they used to do. Things are getting back to how they should be. The numbness will not last forever. The numbness served a purpose – it stopped the pain for a while – it helped you cope. The treatment is over – you no longer have use for the numbness. Just like you no longer need to be numbed by your regrets. It is time to feel and experience new sensations.

*(Guidance note: the hypnotherapist will then work with the client to focus on what they want to feel now the numbness has gone)*

# Chapter 23

# Why I did what I did

## Introduction

An important part of working through regrets is to gain an understanding about how something happened – why the client did or said something. An essential part of the process is to understand what the client was thinking and feeling at the time, that is, the reasoning underpinning the behaviour. Many clients can find it extremely difficult to talk about what they did or said because they feel embarrassed or ashamed. Even though the hypnotherapist has explained about confidentiality, the client may still fear they are going to be judged or there might be repercussions from a disclosure. This is especially true for clients who have:

- Committed a crime
- Been forced into doing something to someone else to prove themselves (e.g. gang initiation)
- Bullied someone. It is not uncommon for adult clients to be racked with guilt about what they did decades ago (e.g. in school).

At times it is difficult to find the right words to talk about or explain something in the conscious state – especially for younger children. It is often so much easier to talk about difficult matters in the trance state and this script is an ideal way of first getting the client into the trance state by watching clouds in the sky and then going back in time to understand why the client behaved as they did.

## The script

Sometimes it is hard to remember things or it is difficult to think about things in the conscious state. It is such a good thing that the subconscious mind protects us – that's its job. So going into trance – being in the hypnotic state can help us remember – help us understand why we behaved as we did – why we said what we said. It could be very true when a person says they can't remember or they don't know why they did something. The subconscious mind may have suppressed the

DOI: 10.4324/9781003468325-27

memory to protect the person. The subconscious mind works best when you are relaxed, so let's get you into a deep, relaxed state.

Imagine that you are in a large loft. There is a bed in the middle of the loft. It is a water bed. Water beds are so comfortable. Go and lie down on the water bed. Feel the water ripple gently underneath your head – your neck – your shoulders – your back – your arms – your hands – your legs – and your feet. Just sink right down into the water bed – feel the water supporting you. Moving gently – swaying. You are starting to feel relaxed – supported – and safe. Supported and safe to remember what you need to remember – to understand why you did what you did – why you said what you said. You are feeling relaxed – supported – and safe.

Now look up at the ceiling. There is a large skylight window and it is propped wide open. You get a clear view of the sky – nothing gets in your way of seeing the sky. Now a lot of people enjoy watching the sun rise at dawn and it certainly is a beautiful time of day. The sunshine brings brightness and hope when a new day is dawning. Another beautiful time of day is the evening. This is what I want you to imagine as you look through the open window.

It is summertime. It stays light until very late into the evening. It takes time for the darkness to come. It is not like in winter when suddenly it is dark – the daylight comes to a sudden end. In the summer months, darkness comes more gently. So look up to the sky. The sky is blue and the sun is still shining. There are some white clouds in the sky, but as it starts to get later in the day the clouds start to change colour. They move and change into all sorts of different shapes in the sky. This is what is so beautiful about this time of year – this time of evening – different colours appear in the sky. The clouds in the sky look white – fluffy – like cotton wool. Maybe you see some bits of blue mixed in with the white. All sorts of different colours can appear within the clouds. Imagine some of the colours now – pink – dark pink – and light pink. Purple mixed with pink. A bit of grey can contrast with the pink and purple. On occasions some bits of orange can appear. It is all so fascinating how different colours can emerge. It is also so relaxing.

The colours appear across the sky within the clouds. The clouds change into different shapes as they move along the sky – the shapes evolve – keep moving. You may see bands of colour in the clouds – across the sky. The clouds look so fluffy and soft – fluffy and soft. Watch the clouds moving along the sky – different shapes evolve – the clouds keep moving. See the colours changing within the clouds. As you look at the clouds and the colours you are becoming more and more relaxed. Watch the clouds – watch the colours – fluffy and soft. So relaxing – you are becoming more and more relaxed.

It would be so lovely to go up into the sky and into those colours. Become even more relaxed. So imagine lifting yourself off the waterbed and floating upwards towards the open window. Keep looking at the colours in the sky. Float upwards and upwards – through the open window – and up and up into the sky. Floating towards the colours – soft and fluffy. You are feeling relaxed and safe. Floating up and up – high into the sky – floating towards the colours.

You are very near the colours now and very soon you are going to float through the colours and go backwards in time. Your subconscious mind is going to take you back in time and help you understand why you did what you did – why you said what you said. There is nothing to fear. You want to understand what happened – why you did what you did – why you said what you said. There is nothing to fear – you need to know. You are feeling relaxed – supported – and safe.

You are getting nearer to the clouds and the colours now. Nearly there – almost there. Now floating through the clouds and the colours – floating back in time. Back to the time when you did what you did – you said what you said. Back and back in time. Remember what happened. Remember what you were thinking. Remember what you were feeling. Remember the reasons you did what you did – you said what you said.

*(Guidance note: the hypnotherapist should then work with the client to talk about what happened and why they regret what they did. Some general questions/ prompts are given below, but every situation is going to be unique so the hypnotherapist may wish to use more specific questions to suit the circumstances)*

Where are you?
When did this happen?
Tell me/describe what is happening.
What happens next?
How are you feeling in this situation?
What was the reason for doing this?
What was the reason for saying this?
What were you thinking then?
What are you thinking now?
What were you feeling then?
What are you feeling now?
What did you do?
What did you say?

Well done for remembering what you did and what you said (*or insert more specific feedback from what has been worked on*). I want you to accept that what happened is in the past and you cannot change what happened, but you can think and feel differently about it. You can accept what happened and you can learn from that experience. People can change and people do change. You are a different person now and you will not act in the same way again. You have felt remorse/regret (*or insert other appropriate words the client has used*) about what you did and what you said and you are doing something positive about that now, which is to be commended.

So now just relax – imagine you are back lying on the water bed looking through the skylight window. Look at the clouds and colours in the sky. The clouds are moving – changing into different shapes – they keep moving – evolving. You are like the clouds – you can keep moving – changing – evolving. You do not have to stay in the same place – be the same person. You can be different – you can change – you can be any way you want to be. You are constantly evolving as you keep moving. Keep watching the clouds – see them change into different shapes as they move along the sky – the shapes evolve – they keep moving. You will keep moving – changing – evolving – won't you?

Chapter 24

# I should have

## Introduction

It is said hindsight is great thing and I agree it often is. It is also said thinking about "what-ifs" is a waste of time. This script encourages the client to reflect back on what they have done and what they regret; and consider what they should have done. A theme throughout this book is that everyone can learn from their past and release the emotions attached to any regrets they may have. The main objective is to work on acknowledgement and acceptance. Regarding some regrets, the client may feel they need to do something in the here and now, i.e. explain to someone why they did what they did. So part of the script works on identifying any actions for Stage 3 of the process.

Using this script encourages the client to think about their regrets and write them down in a notebook. The hypnotherapist can use the forms in Appendices 24.1 and 24.2 to make notes about the regrets and any actions for the future which are identified. However, it is also possible to do the first part of the script as an exercise in the conscious state i.e. identifying the regrets and the "I should have's". Very often when I am working with a client I give them a notebook to use for exercises we might do in a session or when they are at home; for reflective thoughts or to make any notes. In the script the client imagines writing in a notebook; if some of the work is undertaken in the conscious state then the hypnotherapist should have paper or a notebook to hand for the client to use.

## The script

When you are feeling regretful it is very natural to think about what you should have done or what you could have done differently. It is a bit like thinking about "what-ifs". You can find yourself spending too much time thinking about what you should have done. That is not healthy. You know you cannot undo your actions, but it is important to acknowledge what you have done and accept it. Acknowledgement and acceptance are vital to processing your regrets and moving away from them – and moving forward in your life. You need to acknowledge to yourself what

DOI: 10.4324/9781003468325-28

you have done and in some circumstances it may be helpful to tell or explain to someone else what you have done. Yes you are talking to me now but I wonder if you need to tell anyone else – someone who is perhaps connected to the regrets. So for now talk to me. Let us think about what you should have done and then work towards acknowledgment and acceptance.

I want you to imagine that you are in a room and sitting at a desk. The desk is clear – nothing on it all. Clear like your mind is becoming as you focus on your regrets. Your mind is becoming clearer and clearer. Open one of the drawers in the desk and you will find a brand new notebook and pen. On the front of the notebook you will see the words "I should have". Open the book and then flick through it. You will see that all the pages are new and unused. Go back to the first page and write the word "Contents" at the top of the page. You are going to write down and number the regrets you have been reflecting on recently. First of all, just sit back and think about your regrets for a while before you start writing. When you are ready start writing them down – make a list – number the regrets. Tell me when you have finished writing the list.

*(Guidance note: the form in Appendix 24.1 is provided for the hypnotherapist to use with this script)*

In a moment I want you to read through the list again. It may be for some of the regrets you have listed at some time previously you have thought "I should have". This might not be the case for every regret you have written down, so I want you to read slowly through the list again and tell me if you have ever thought "I should have" in relation to a particular regret. Take your time.

*(Guidance note: if/when the client does identify a "I should have" regret the following questions can be used to get more detail)*

Tell me more about the actual regret.
What do you think you should have done?
Did you think about doing that at the time? If yes, what was the reason for not doing that?
Do you think it would have made a difference?

You need to accept that you did not (*insert the "I should have"*). You cannot change that. Acknowledge it now and accept that it is not healthy to dwell on the past and what might have happened if you had done something differently. It is important for your health and wellbeing to focus on the here and now – and the way forward. To do that think about whether you need to tell or explain to anyone about what you did do and how you feel about that now. Is there anything you need to do? Is there anyone you need to speak with?

*(Guidance note: the hypnotherapist should allow the client to think about any action(s) they may want to take before proceeding with questions to get detailed information about what the client wants to do)*

So what would you like to do?
When will you do this?
When will you have done this by?

*(Guidance note: the form in Appendix 24.2 can be used to plan the action and set a timescale if appropriate. After helping the client to plan their action, the hypnotherapist will check if there are any other "I should have's" and then repeat the process)*

Look at your notebook again. Are there any more regrets listed where you have thought "I should have"?

Well done – you have faced the past and thought about what you should have done. You have also considered whether you need to take action now. Remember you cannot change what you did not do. Acknowledge it now and accept that it is not healthy to dwell on the past and what might have happened if you had done something differently. It is important for your health and wellbeing to focus on the here and now – and the way forward – and that is what you are going to do now – over the next few days, weeks and months. Say out loud to yourself: I shall ...

*(Guidance note: the hypnotherapist can summarise the actions the client has identified)*

## Appendix 24.1: Form for identifying the "I should have's"

## *I SHOULD HAVE*

Name of client:                                   Date of session:

1.  The regret identified:
    Is there an "I should have" attached to the regret?       Yes  [ ]   No [ ]
    If yes, give detail about this:

2.  The regret identified:
    Is there an "I should have" attached to the regret?       Yes  [ ]   No [ ]
    If yes, give detail about this:

3.  The regret identified:
    Is there an "I should have" attached to the regret?       Yes  [ ]   No [ ]
    If yes, give detail about this:

4.  The regret identified:
    Is there an "I should have" attached to the regret?       Yes  [ ]   No [ ]
    If yes, give detail about this:

5.  The regret identified:
    Is there an "I should have" attached to the regret?       Yes  [ ]   No [ ]
    If yes, give detail about this:

## Appendix 24.2: Form for actions to be taken

### *ACTIONS*

Name of client:                                    Date of session:

**<u>Action</u>**                    **<u>What needs to be done</u>**                    **<u>Timescale</u>**

Chapter 25

# Fear of failing

## Introduction

We are encouraged to be successful from a very early age. A lot of pressure is put on both children and adults to succeed. I actually think this has got worse in recent decades; especially for children who in infant school have to be tested and life becomes very competitive even in that early stage. Regrets are often linked to a sense of having failed and a fear can develop that it is going to happen again. This fear of failing can result in a loss of confidence and low self-esteem. Clients often say "I feel like a failure" and believe other people see them as such.

It is essential for a client to understand that failing is a part of life and part of the learning curve that everyone travels long. Some failures will not be significant; when they happen it will not seem like the end of the world. Other failures may have more impact on how a person thinks, feels and behaves over time. This script aims to create a positive attitude and to see that lessons can be learnt from failing. It can be useful to repeat the script in each session.

I use this script for both children and adults. Children can struggle with learning and/or studying due to having a problem with concentration/focussing (as can adults) and feel they are failing because they are not academic. I do not think it helps when parents are pushing a child too hard and teachers are also emphasising over and over again the importance of exams. There are ways of getting the message across and encouraging a child without making a big thing out of it – so much so it creates fear in the child. The fear of failing as stated above can result in a loss of confidence, but it can also result in exam anxiety (and panic attacks). Every human being is good at something – and it might not necessarily be at academic subjects. Adults can look back and wish they had tried harder (i.e. that is the regret) because a lot of jobs require particular qualifications they have not got. They can believe that they failed at school or college, but in fact they have been very successful in other aspects of their life, where they have developed practical skills. However, they fail to acknowledge what they have succeeded in doing – perhaps because of having low self-esteem.

At the end of the script I have inserted a list of questions which the hypnotherapist can use to undertake more in-depth work with the client. The form in Appendix

DOI: 10.4324/9781003468325-29

25.1 can be used to take detailed notes about specific fears the client has in regard to failing.

## The script

There are words in our language that sound so harsh. As soon as you hear them you can feel a negative emotion. Failure is one such word. I wonder how you felt when I said that word – failure. Failure is the opposite of success. From a young age you are expected to succeed. New mums compare how their babies are developing and feel they themselves are failing if their baby is not doing what another baby is doing (e.g. crawling, getting a first tooth, walking). From a very young age you will have become aware of success and failure. Think of experiences at school – passing or failing tests and exams. Students are expected to meet certain standards to succeed – GCSEs, A levels to get to college or university. Perhaps you went for trials to get into some team (*insert as appropriate from knowledge about the client or use e.g. football; netball*) or you have auditioned for something (*e.g. a choir; a band; a play; a musical*). From a very early age you are put under pressure to succeed and life can be competitive – comparisons being made again and again.

So let's change the way you think and feel about failure – and ultimately this will affect the way you will behave in the future. I often say to clients a positive can always come out of a negative. Similarly, lessons can be learnt from failing to do something – this can be a positive. It is all too easy to always focus on the negatives rather than the positives. This can become a habit. The consequence can be that you develop a fear of failing. As this fear grows you can lose your confidence and you do not believe in yourself. You think you are going to fail again. This can result in not trying for certain things – playing it safe. You write your own script – you predict failure and you make it happen. You can then become obsessed with focusing on the past and failing – your failings. You actually set yourself up to fail. You predict failure. It becomes a self-fulfilling prophecy. If this happens, it is important to change the way you think and change the way you feel. You need to change the way you think and feel about failure. Instead you need to focus on the lessons learnt from a failure – so the failure has a positive outcome for the future. Everyone is good at something – not one human being in this world can be good at absolutely everything. It is essential to identify and focus on your attributes – your knowledge – your skills – and to use them to your greatest benefit.

*(Guidance note: below are some questions to facilitate work on identifying what the client thinks they have failed at, when this happened and what lessons they have learnt from the failure. It is best to identify the main failures first and then to talk about each one separately. A form is presented in Appendix 25.1 for the hypnotherapist to use as this work is undertaken)*

What do you think has been the main/significant failures in your lifetime?
When have you failed?

Tell me about one particular failure.

What makes you think you failed?

Did anyone else think you had failed?

Did anyone tell you that you had failed? If yes, Who said this? What did they say exactly? What did you think about what they said?

Did they say it more than once?

How did that make you feel?

How did you react?

Did you think you had failed at the time?

What was the reason for thinking that?

Looking back now, do you still think you failed?

How did the failure affect you in the past?

Does the failure affect you now? If yes, In what way?

How did you feel when you failed?

How long did these feelings last?

Did your behaviour change in any way? If yes, how did it change?

How often do you think about this failure?

What lessons have you learnt from this failure?

Could you have done anything differently?

What would you say to (*name of client*) back then?

What would you say to (*name of client*) now?

*(Guidance note: if the client identifies more than one failure, the above questions can be repeated to gain the detail/information. The process will be repeated for each failure identified)*

You now accept that failing at something is not necessarily a bad or negative thing – it can be a good and positive thing because you can learn from the experience and use it to your benefit in the future. You know that you can change the way you think and change the way you feel about what has happened in the past and you are capable of achieving great things in the future. Believe in yourself. Have confidence in yourself. Everyone is good at something – not one human being in this world can be good at absolutely everything. It is essential to identify and focus on your attributes – your knowledge – your skills – and to use them for your greatest benefit. And you will won't you?

## Appendix 25.1: Form for recording failings and failures identified

### *FAILINGS AND FAILURES IDENTIFIED*

Name of client:                                     Date:

| Date/year | Detail/information | Lessons learnt |
|-----------|-------------------|----------------|
| 1. | | |
| 2. | | |
| 3. | | |
| 4. | | |
| 5. | | |
| 6. | | |
| 7. | | |
| 8. | | |
| 9. | | |
| 10. | | |

Chapter 26

# Street art

## Introduction

This script should be used with a client who finds it difficult to express themselves verbally in the conscious state; or with any client who enjoys drawing, painting or being creative in general. The idea is to get the client to express the emotions associated with their regrets by painting street art on electricity power cabinets, but also to embed that they are in control and have the power to surge forward.

## The script

Some people find it hard in general to express their feelings. Maybe they are shy – or maybe they are very private and do not want people to know their business – or maybe they just cannot find the right words. Other people may find certain things hard to talk about. So it can be helpful to find other ways of expressing oneself – other ways of expressing your emotions – by writing – by drawing – by painting in your imagination. I know you have been struggling a bit to talk about how you have been feeling in relation to the regrets you have, so let us see what we can do about that.

I want you to imagine that you are in a city – a city in your mind. Imagine walking along the streets – looking all around you. Look at the people – the buildings – the traffic. Be observant – look all around you. You can learn so much from being observant – watching closely – listening closely.

In this city there is a lot of street art. Some of it is on walls – some of it is on the side of buildings – and some of it is on the electricity power cabinets that you see on the streets, which are often green or grey in colour. Keep exploring the city and watch out for the street art. Tell me what you see. Tell me when you see something that interests you. What street art are you seeing?

*(Guidance note: it often happens that the client brings forward what has been on their mind or troubling them. If this happens, it is important for the hypnotherapist to discuss this in as much detail as possible)*

DOI: 10.4324/9781003468325-30

Tell me about the street art you are seeing.
Where is it painted exactly?
What are you seeing in the street art?
How does the street art make you feel?
Do you think there is a message in the street art?
Is the anything you would like to change in what you are seeing?

*(Guidance note: if the client would like to change something the hypnotherapist will encourage them to paint the changes)*

What do you want to change?
What do you want to be different?
What changes will you make?

Find some paint and paintbrushes and make those changes now. Tell me what you are doing as you paint.

Now I want you to find a street where there is an electricity power cabinet. The cabinet will be just one colour – either green or grey. Tell me when you have found it. Around the cabinet you will see lots of tins of paint – both big and small – and there are so many different colours – you can use whatever you like. There will also be different sized paintbrushes for you to use. Just sit in front of the cabinet for a minute. You see just one colour – green or grey. Think about your regrets. Bring forward the emotions you have been experiencing in relation to your regrets. Maybe you are thinking about just one emotion – maybe there are lots of emotions flooding through. Concentrate on your emotions – bring them forward – do not fear them – rather feel them. Really feel them.

Now I want you to paint on the cabinet. Paint what you feel. You have lots of paint to choose from – all different colours. Start painting – paint your emotions. Describe to me what you are painting as you create your street art.

*(Guidance note: the hypnotherapist will engage with the client as they paint. It will be important to understand what is being created and how the client is feeling as they do it. Some questions below can be used if required)*

What are you creating?
What is in the street art?
Are you putting in any people? If yes, who are they?
What else are you putting in?
What colours are you using?
How is it coming along?
How are you feeling as you create your street art?
What are you thinking about as you create your street art?
Tell me when you have finished creating your street art.

Now stand back – away from the electricity power cabinet. Look at the street art you have created.

What does it tell you?
Is there a message in the street art?
How do you feel now you have created this piece of street art?
Do you need to create another piece of street art?

*(Guidance note: there will be times when the client only needs to draw one piece of street art to depict all the emotions. However, some clients want to create more street art on different electricity power cabinets. If this is the case, the hypnotherapist should take the client to another street to find another cabinet and create another piece of street art)*

Well done you have created some wonderful street art that tells a story – the story about your emotions – how you have been feeling in relation to your regrets. Now I want you to focus on *(or one of the)* the electricity power cabinet*(s)* you have painted. Look at the street art again painted on the cabinet. Now think about the power inside the cabinet. Open the door of the cabinet and look inside – you may see some wires but there are lots of other things too – switches – levers – knobs – dials – display units – which are all part of the control system. The power is there – safe and protected – ready to surge forward whenever it is needed. Imagine the power – imagine the surge. Feel the power – feel the surge.

You have the power to control your emotions. You can control how you feel about your regrets. You can switch the regrets on and off. You can switch your emotions on and off. You can switch your thoughts on and off. You have so many things you can use in the cabinet – wiring – switches – levers – knobs – dials – display units – which are all part of the control system. So maybe you would like to switch something off now. What would you like to switch off? Use a switch and do that now. You can turn your emotions up and down. Turn down a negative emotion. Turn up a positive emotion. What would you like to do? Use a lever and do that now. You have all these tools to help you in the electricity power cabinet. You are in complete control. You have the power – you are safe and protected – you can surge forward at any time. You have the power to surge forward. Do that now – turn your power on and surge forward.

# Part V

# Taking action

# Chapter 27

# Let's think about the Rs

## Introduction

This script should be used when work has been done to identify the regrets and the client has already done some initial talking around their thoughts and feelings. The objective of the script is for the client to think more deeply about their regrets by focusing on the letter R, which they climb and walk around to reflect and review. The client thinks about what needs to be done in order to make them feel better i.e. release the emotions associated with the regrets or to take some particular action. This script will help to plan the work which needs to be done in the future and can be used in conjunction with other scripts presented in Part V.

## The script

R is for regrets. The regrets you have identified and acknowledged – the regrets we have been discussing. I want you to visualise the letter R. Look at the letter – sense that it is in front of you. R is for regrets, but R can be for many other things too. Let's think about this. Consider the letter R. A big capital R. See it in front of you. Then imagine you are standing at the bottom of the letter R. Look up at the huge letter. You are going to start to climb the letter R. I wonder which end you will start from. I wonder if you will you go up the straight back of the R – over the top – and then down the other side. Or maybe you will start by going up the slanting bit of the R first – over the top – and then down the other side. It really does not matter – it is completely up to you. It will be a steep climb whichever way you go. So when you are ready – *1, 2,* and *3* – start climbing and think about the regrets you have been talking about.

R can be for regrets. R can be for reflection. R can be for review. Reflecting back and reviewing what happened – what was done or not done – what was said or not said. Reflecting back and reviewing can be a really good thing to do. It can bring some understanding and some clarity about what has already happened but it can also bring some understanding and clarity about what needs to be done now and in the future. So keep climbing up the letter R and walk around it. Walk around the R – reflecting and reviewing. Reflect on your regrets. Review your regrets. Walk

DOI: 10.4324/9781003468325-32

around the R – take your time – there is no need to rush. It is a steep climb – so remember to take some deep breaths in and out as you climb up and up – over the top – and down and down. Reflecting and reviewing. Keep walking. Tell me when you have finished walking around the R.

Good – take some deep breaths before you climb and walk around the R again. Before you reflect and review again. Take some more deep breaths. You are going to climb and walk around the R several times now. Reflecting and reviewing. Climbing up the R will get easier the more times you do it. I am going to be quiet for a while so you can keep climbing and walking around the R – reflecting and reviewing again. Go around the R as many times as you want – reflecting and reviewing. Tell me when you have finished reflecting and reviewing. Take as much time as you need. Now tell me what you have been reflecting on and what you have been reviewing.

*(Guidance note: the hypnotherapist should allow time for discussion)*

Now climb to the top of the R again and when you reach the top sit and make yourself comfortable. I want you to start thinking about other words that begin with the letter R and are relevant or significant for your regrets. What words are coming forward?

I am reflecting now about some words clients have said to me when thinking about what they need to stop feeling regretful. Not all the words will be relevant to your regrets, but some may help you think about what you need to do, say or explain – or what you need to ask other people to do, say or explain. So reflect on these words:

| | |
|---|---|
| • Remorse | • Reward |
| • Repent | • Reassert |
| • Rectify | • Recharge |
| • Return | • Restore |
| • Reconcile | • Revive |
| • Reconnect | • Release. |
| • Repay | |

Let me repeat those words for you to reflect on:

| | |
|---|---|
| • Remorse | • Reward |
| • Repent | • Reassert |
| • Rectify | • Recharge |
| • Return | • Restore |
| • Reconcile | • Revive |
| • Reconnect | • Release. |
| • Repay | |

What have any of those words made you think about?
How do any of those words make you feel?
What have those words brought forward in your mind?
Are any of those words relevant to your regrets?
Are any other words beginning with R coming forward now?

You know it is important to think about your regrets – it is just as important to work through them and that might involve taking some action. Ask yourself if you need to do anything in relation to your regrets. Do you need to take any action? Reflect on that for a short time while you take another walk around the R. Do you need to take any action? If you need to walk around the R several times that is fine. Just tell me when you have finished reflecting.

What have you been reflecting on?
Do you need to take any action?
What do you want to do?
What do you want to say?
Do you need to do, say or explain anything to anyone?
What do you need to do?
What do you need to say?
What do you need to explain?
Does anyone else need to do, say or explain anything to you?
What do you want to know?
What do you need to find out?

*(Guidance note: the hypnotherapist and client should identify what action
needs to be taken and then in future sessions the action can be planned in
detail using scripts from Part V. The hypnotherapist might find it useful
for recording purposes to use the form presented in Appendix 24.2 to list
the actions discussed)*

# Chapter 28

# It's never too late

## Introduction

This is a good script to use when a client is starting to plan some action in regard to their regrets (Stage 3), but it can be used at any point during a treatment plan which is focused on working through regrets. I believe it is good to use the script more than once when working with a client on their regrets. It embeds the idea that it is never too late to do something about a regret, which may require taking action in regard to a situation, a relationship, something that happened a long time ago or even more recently. As already discussed in earlier chapters, all sorts of regrets could be presented to the hypnotherapist and consequently there could be a vast number of actions that could help resolve a situation. The possibilities are endless.

So this script is a gentle starting point to encourage the client to accept that it is never too late to take action and not to give up. Many clients present as feeling resigned that nothing can be done – this script aims to embed a positive attitude that something can be done. Other scripts should then be used to identify actions which need to be undertaken.

The title of the script can also be used as a mantra. I use mantras a lot with my clients, so I have included a very short additional script at the end to introduce the mantra – It's never too late.

## The script

I know that you may feel that it is too late to do anything about (*insert regret(s) discussed previously*), but the truth is it is never too late. It is never too late to do something about the way you think – the way you feel – the way you behave. It is never too late to take action – make changes – speak out – explain – find the truth – make amends. I want you to relax deeper now so that you can think about this. Your subconscious mind works better when you are relaxing – when you relax both your body and mind. So go deeper now – deeper and deeper into the trance state.

I wonder if you have ever thought about how often we are told that because we are a certain age we should not do something or we should have done or achieved something by this stage in our life. You will have been told you are too young or too old to do something. Right from childhood we are made aware of age – timing

DOI: 10.4324/9781003468325-33

– what is acceptable and what is not acceptable. There is such an emphasis on age – being age appropriate. We are influenced by society's expectations from the moment we are born. Just think of some the things you have heard people say so often. You are on the shelf if you have not been married by a certain age. The disdain in someone's voice when they refer to someone as being a spinster. It is often intimated that time is running out. A woman being told she is too old to have a baby. What is being old exactly? A government in a country defines it by retirement age. People who want to work beyond state retirement age are often asked frequently when they are going to retire and thought to be odd if they want to carry on working. So what is old age – age 55, 60, 66, 70, 80 or 90 – who knows? There are different claims about who has been the oldest person to live in the world – a 122-year-old woman in France – another woman aged 128 years in Dominica – and a man allegedly was 157 years old when he died in Turkey. So if living to any of these ages became the norm being 50 years old would not even be middle-aged. So the cliché is true – age is just a number. Nevertheless, we are made to think about age and timing and this can result in thinking it is too late to do something, but it is never too late. It is never too late to take action – make changes – speak out – explain – find the truth – make amends.

Let's think about this a little bit more as you go deeper and deeper into trance. Think about – it's never too late. Accept that it is never too late to take action – make changes – speak out – explain – find the truth – make amends. And you will accept that won't you? You have come for therapy in order to work on your regrets. The fact that you are here shows that you have not given up – you want to take action – you want to make some changes. You know that you can change the way you think – the way you feel – and the way you behave. You are doing that right now. You have the motivation and you have the determination. You accept that it is never too late – never too late to do something about what is bothering you. Your regrets have been bothering you and now it is time to do something about it – and you will won't you?

*(Guidance note: if the hypnotherapist would like to introduce the idea of using a mantra the following additional script can be used. Otherwise another script should be used to follow on and identify exactly what needs to be worked on)*

## Additional script: Optional mantra

Focus now on those words: It's never too late. Say them to yourself silently: It's never too late. And again to yourself: It's never too late. Now say those words out loud: It's never too late. And again – louder this time: It's never too late. And louder: It's never too late. You believe in those words: It's never too late. So as you accept and believe in those words – let those words become a mantra for you while you take action over the next few days, weeks and months: It's never too late. Every day you will say to yourself silently or out loud: It's never too late. Say it to yourself when you wake up – when you are in the house – when you are outside – when you at work – and before you go to sleep: It's never too late. Because it never is too late, is it?

# Chapter 29

# The meeting room

## Introduction

The purpose of the script is to enable the client to set up a meeting room where they can prepare and plan their actions before meeting with or confronting someone. The meeting room is a place where they can rehearse what they are going to say and do if they are going to have conversations which may be difficult. The idea is that the client can come back to the room as often as they like and rehearse what they are going to say and do.

The script was written to prepare for face-to-face meetings, but it can be adapted if the client is going to communicate by phone or perhaps online via Zoom, Skype etc.

A very short additional script is presented to embed the idea that confrontation can be a positive thing. The word is often associated with negativity, when in fact confronting someone in a calm and confident manner can bring positive outcomes and resolution to a situation.

It is helpful to use the main script to set up the meeting room and then use the script in the following chapter to focus the client on communication skills and how they should present themselves when they meet with someone.

## The script

You have spent time thinking about your regrets and you have done some excellent work acknowledging them and realising how they have affected you. Now it is time to take some action. You know what you need to do (*insert what has been discussed and agreed*). It is never a good idea to act in haste or to rush things. It is much better to think – plan – prepare – and then rehearse. That can be a helpful mantra – think – plan – prepare – rehearse. Remember – think – plan – prepare – rehearse. You need to feel calm and relaxed when you do this. You need to have a place where you can plan your actions – what you want to do – what you want to say – what you want to find out. Your subconscious mind works so well when you are feeling calm and relaxed.

DOI: 10.4324/9781003468325-34

So you are going to imagine a room – a meeting room – where you can think – plan – prepare – rehearse. It will be a place you can visit as often as you wish to do so. Now just relax – slow your breathing down. You know how to do this so well. Slow it right down. You are feeling calm – even calmer now – slow your breathing down even more. Relax your mind – calm your mind. If your mind drifts that is absolutely fine. You are feeling really calm and relaxed now.

On the count of *3*, you will see the meeting room – *1, 2,* and *3*. You are in the meeting room. A place where you can you can think – plan – prepare – rehearse. You feel calm and relaxed in here so you can achieve whatever needs to be done. Look around the room – see what furniture and equipment is in the room. What do you see? You can bring in anything you might need for the work you are going to do. It is important to feel good when you are working. You need your strength – so maybe you might want to bring in some food or drink for sustenance. Tell me more about this meeting room and what you need in it to think – plan – prepare – rehearse.

*(Guidance note: usually a client has no problem at all in creating their meeting room and the hypnotherapist should not be surprised if odd things are brought into the room e.g. a fridge, cooker, television etc. However, if this is not the case – or if the hypnotherapist plans to use a particular script which requires a certain object/facility – the client can be asked if they need or to bring any of the following into the meeting room:*

- *Desk/table*
- *Filing cabinet*
- *Waste paper bin*
- *Paper shredder*
- *Television*
- *Computer/laptop*
- *Printer*
- *Mobile/telephone)*

Now I want you to think about the actions you are going to take – what you need to plan for. You have talked about (*insert what has been agreed i.e. who the client is going to meet/have a conversation with*). Why not sit down – make yourself comfortable – and just think about what needs to be done. Maybe you would like to think about the practical things first:

Where would be a good place to meet?
What is a convenient time to meet?
How long do you think you will need for this meeting/conversation?

Now think about what you want to get from this meeting – what you want the outcome to be. Then you can plan how you are going to do this. Remember think – plan – prepare – rehearse.

*(Guidance note: the following questions can be used as a starting point to get the client to think about what they actually want to talk about)*

What do you want to say?
What do you need to explain?
What do you want to ask?
What do you need to know?
What do you want the outcome to be?

When you are going to meet with someone to discuss something important you need to decide where and how you want to be. Are you are going to sit or stand? Ensure there is sufficient distance between you and remove any barriers. Nobody should hide behind a desk or table – a computer or laptop screen – or be doing something else – like checking their mobile phone – so they are not giving you their full attention.

Now visualise where the meeting will take place. Tell me who is in the room. Tell me what happens.

What do you say exactly?
How does (*person*) react?
What does (*person*) say?
How do you react?
How do you respond?
How are you feeling?
What do you say next?

*(Guidance note: time will be spent planning the meeting/conversation and this may need to be done over several sessions by coming back to the meeting room to rehearse. It is important to do some ego boosting at the end of each session)*

## Additional script: Confrontation can be a positive thing

Many people do not like the word "confrontation". They can think it sounds aggressive and makes them feel uncomfortable. This is probably due to the fact that definitions of confrontation often include the words – hostile – argumentative – conflict – battle – opposition – demonstration – all of which are negative. Confrontation does not have to be a negative thing. Confrontation does not have to be something to fear or dread. Confrontation can be a positive thing. Confrontation is about facing a person or situation. It is about being – honest – transparent – up front – talking about what you think – talking about what you feel – talking about what you want to happen. Confrontation can result in positive outcomes – getting answers – finding out the truth – making changes. Confrontation can be undertaken in a calm – confident – assertive – non-aggressive manner. You can do this. You can confront someone (*or insert name of person*) in a calm – confident – assertive – non-aggressive manner and then you will achieve what you want from that confrontation. Confrontation can bring solutions and resolution. Confrontation can be a positive thing.

# Chapter 30

# Communication and presenting oneself

## Introduction

A client may decide that they need to have a meeting with someone which might involve having to have a difficult conversation. It is useful to spend a whole session focusing on good communication skills (both listening and responding), which should involve working on body language. Preparation and rehearsal are vital in order to build confidence. This script helps the client to consider their own body language, which will include body positioning and movement, voice, eye contact, facial expressions and breathing, by bringing forward past situations and reframing. Depending on the length of the session, the script may take up a whole session and a separate session may be needed to rehearse a particular situation for the future.

## The script

I think it might be helpful if we spend some time thinking about how to present yourself when you meet (*insert name of person*). Our bodies do all sorts of things when we are feeling worried, nervous, apprehensive or fearful. Sometimes we do not even notice what our body is doing, but the person we are communicating with might pick up on some clues from our body language. You know that preparation, rehearsal and practice are important. Today I want us to work on communication and think about how to present yourself when you meet (*insert name of person*). Now your body is made up of lots of different parts and you need to be thinking about all of them.

I want us to work on – body positioning and movement – your voice – eye contact – facial expressions – and breathing. Now you know a lot about breathing already, so let us start with that and get you nice and relaxed. Let's do some number breathing first of all. Let's breathe in for *3* and then out for *3*. Ready ...

Breathe in: *1, 2, 3* – and hold
Breathe out: *3, 2, 1* – relax. And again.
Breathe in: *1, 2, 3* – and hold

DOI: 10.4324/9781003468325-35

Breathe out: *3, 2, 1* – relax. One more time.
Breathe in: *1, 2, 3* – and hold
Breathe out: *3, 2, 1* – relax. Good. Feeling relaxed and calm.

Now let's go to *4*.

Breathe in: *1, 2, 3, 4* – and hold
Breathe out: *4, 3, 2, 1* – relax. And again.
Breathe in: *1, 2, 3, 4* – and hold
Breathe out: *4, 3, 2, 1* – relax. One more time.
Breathe in: *1, 2, 3, 4* – and hold
Breathe out: *4, 3, 2, 1* – relax.

Now let's try some ratio breathing – let's try *2* and *4* first of all.

Breathe in: *1* and *2*
Breathe out: *4, 3, 2,* and *1* – and again.
Breathe in: *1* and *2*
Breathe out: *4, 3, 2,* and *1* – and again.
Breathe in: *1* and *2*
Breathe out: *4, 3, 2,* and 1 – good – well done.

Now let's try *3* and *6*.

Breathe in: *1, 2* and *3*
Breathe out: *6, 5, 4, 3, 2* and *1*.
Breathe in: *1, 2* and *3*
Breathe out: *6, 5, 4, 3, 2* and *1*. One more time.
Breathe in: *1, 2* and *3*
Breathe out: *6, 5, 4, 3, 2* and *1*.

Good – you are nice and relaxed now. Enjoy feeling relaxed. You know you can feel like this by breathing nice and slowly. It is such a simple thing to do and you know already how beneficial it is to practise your breathing several times a day. So when you experience any nervousness or any other negative feeling you will remember to breathe. Take a moment and breathe. Take a breath and breathe. Breathe nice and slowly. Never be rushed or feel forced to speak or react immediately to what has been said. Take a moment and breathe. Take a breath and breathe. Breathe nice and slowly.

I want you to think back to any situations and the places you were in when you have felt worried, nervous, apprehensive or fearful. Just let your mind drift back to those situations and places. Look at yourself in those situations and places. Look at where you are standing or sitting. Is there enough space between you and other people? Are there any physical objects or obstacles in the way? Focus now on your body. Notice whether you are still or whether you are swaying. I wonder if some parts of your body are moving about. Look at your hands and feet. Are you fiddling with something? Is a leg moving up and down or a foot jogging? I wonder if you are fidgeting at all. Keep thinking back to any situations and the places you were in when you have felt worried, nervous, apprehensive or fearful. Just let your mind drift back to those situations and places. Look at yourself in those situations and places.

*(Guidance note: the hypnotherapist should be silent so the client can think about the situations before focusing on one particular situation)*

Now I want you to focus on just one of those situations when you were feeling worried, nervous, apprehensive or fearful. Be in that situation again now. Look at yourself in that situation and the place where you are. Look at where you are standing or sitting. Is there enough space between you and other people? Are there any physical objects or obstacles in the way? Focus now on your body. Notice whether you are still or whether you are swaying. I wonder if some parts of your body are moving about. Look at your hands and feet. Are you fiddling with something? Is a leg moving up and down or a foot jogging? I wonder if you are fidgeting at all.

Now imagine how still you can be – not rigid – just still. Still and calm. When you are still you do not have to be rigid or stiff – just relax. Now imagine yourself standing up somewhere. Look at yourself. Notice whether you are still or whether you are moving about. I wonder if some parts of your body are moving about. See how still you can be. Still and calm. When you are still you do not have to be rigid or stiff – just relax. Look closely – see that your body is relaxed – still and calm – still and calm. Look at your chest – look at how you are breathing – nice and slowly – steadily.

Now think about your voice. I wonder what happens to your voice when you feel nervous. Do you stutter – talk too fast – become too quiet so you have to repeat what you have said or does your voice become high-pitched? Think about what happens to your voice when you are worried, nervous, apprehensive or fearful. Think about a situation when you have felt worried, nervous, apprehensive or fearful and your voice was affected. Describe the situation and tell me what happened.

*(Guidance note: the hypnotherapist will discuss this in depth with the client and reframe)*

Now look at that situation again. Listen to your voice. Your voice is a very powerful tool. How you use it can be very effective. You know you can control your voice. First of all I want you to think about what you actually want to say – think about the words you will use. Now focus on your voice – the tone of your voice (calm – relaxed – confident) – the pitch (not too high – not too low) – the volume (not too loud – not too quiet) and the pace at which you speak (not too fast – not too slow).

Who would have thought that there is such a lot to think about in regard to your voice? So give it some more thought – focus on your voice – and make any necessary changes you need:

The tone of your voice: What do you want it to sound like?
The pitch: Does it need to be higher or lower?
The volume: Is it too loud or too quiet?
The pace at which you speak: Do you need to slow down or speed up?

Always speak clearly and remember to put some emphasis on important words to make your meaning clear. Remember you never have to rush – take your time.

Now we need to think about the use of pauses and silences. It can be so easy to rush in with a comment when there is a gap in the conversation. It can feel like you need to fill the silence. I wonder how many times you do rush in. Your breathing will come in useful again here. Take a breath and pause. Take another breath and pause. This gives you thinking time. Take a breath and pause. Take another breath and pause. You may even want to count some seconds before you rush in. A pause can be up to 15 seconds. A silence could be up to a minute. During that time your body needs to remain relaxed. Count some seconds now – count up to 15 seconds. Start counting from *1* – out loud – now.

*(Guidance note: if the client counts quickly the hypnotherapists needs to interject and slow them down and tell them to start from 1 again)*

Do that again now. Count up to 15 seconds.

Well done. Remember that is just a pause. A silence could be up to a minute. So I am going to be silent for a whole minute. I want you to count from *1* upwards to yourself in silence – counting the seconds. You will keep counting until I tell you to stop. You are going to count from *1* upwards – just count nice and slowly – concentrate on your breathing whilst you are counting. Ready to begin – start counting from *1* in silence – now.

*(Guidance note: the hypnotherapist should be silent for exactly a minute and will need to use a watch/timer to do this)*

Stop counting now. So what number did you get to?

*(Guidance note: if the client has gone over 60, then the hypnotherapist should have a discussion about counting slowly and repeat the exercise)*

Well done. Now you have something else to practise – counting for pauses and silences – enjoying pauses and silences. You can practise counting when you are relaxing in the trance state or in the conscious state. Just slow down your counting and slow down your breathing.

Now think about your eyes. When you are speaking with someone or when you are pausing in a conversation it is important to maintain eye contact. No – you are not going to glare or stare at someone. You will look at the person directly and occasionally look away for a second. So you are not staring. Even if the other person looks away from you or refuses to have eye contact with you, you will continue looking at them. You give that person your full attention. Think back to a situation in the past when you know you felt awkward and avoided eye contact. Describe the situation and tell me what happened.

*(Guidance note: the hypnotherapist will discuss this in depth with the client and reframe)*

So we know that it is important that your voice – that very powerful tool – conveys the right message; but it is also important that your face gives the right message too. You need to keep asking yourself the question: "What is my face showing?" There will be times when people will try to bait you – or they will make you angry – or perhaps sad. When a person does not listen to what you say you can feel frustrated. You need to be thinking about your face. You need to remain still and calm – relaxed. Think back to a situation in the past when you know your face showed what you were thinking or feeling – anger, annoyance, frustration, embarrassment or upset. Describe the situation and tell me what happened.

*(Guidance note: the hypnotherapist will discuss this in depth with the client and reframe)*

There is so much to think about in relation to how you present yourself – body positioning and movement – your voice – eye contact – facial expressions – and all the while focusing on your breathing. Over the next few days you will be more aware of all these things – in the conscious state and when you are in the trance state. Being in trance is a good place to be to reflect – observe – rehearse and practise. You are going to become a better communicator because you will be aware of – body positioning and movement – your voice – eye contact – facial expressions – and breathing. Every day you will become more and more confident in how you present yourself – and you yourself will notice these changes when in the conscious state and other people are going to notice how much more confident and assertive you have become.

# Chapter 31

# Your own channel

## Introduction

This script works well for anyone who enjoys watching things on YouTube. It should be used when the client has identified what they need to do i.e. take some action, but maybe is nervous, apprehensive or has reservations about going ahead with it (e.g. meeting someone). The client has their own app and then produces videos to rehearse what they need to do or say when they are in a particular situation (Option 1) or they can talk about/vent how they are feeling or about a certain situation/their regrets (Option 2). It is a script which can be used numerous times so the client creates a library of videos they can revisit and edit if necessary.

## The script

Imagine that your phone is in your hand. Look at the screen and open it up. Start scrolling through the apps because I want you to find a new app which you will see there. It will be called (*insert client's name*)'s Tube. Yes this is your very own app for watching and making videos. It is an app that you can use to be creative – think – plan – prepare – rehearse – watch – and learn. So keep scrolling and tell me when you have found the app. Good. Now open (*insert client's name*)'s Tube. This is going to be so useful to you.

Before you start using (*insert client's name*)'s Tube I just want you to relax – go into a deeper state of trance. You know your subconscious mind works so well when you are relaxed. You can become more and more creative. You can think – plan – prepare – rehearse – watch – and learn. You can (*insert anything that needs to be worked on for the client e.g. confidence*). Just relax now – go deeper and deeper.

As you are becoming more and more relaxed think about (*insert what the client needs to do/what they are worried about e.g. meeting someone; having a conversation*). With (*insert client's name*)'s Tube you could create all sorts of videos. I wonder what you might to do – maybe plan (*insert as appropriate*) or talk about what you think and how you feel. You are safe here – you can try out anything using (*insert client's name*)'s Tube. If something does not feel right or if something

DOI: 10.4324/9781003468325-36

does not sound right – you can pause – you can edit – stop – delete and start again. You can experiment – remake – until everything is just as you want it to be. So what do you want to create?

## Option 1: Preparing for a meeting/conversation

Now it is time to make the video about the meeting (*insert as appropriate*). You are the creator. It is always good to plan and prepare before going to a meeting. It is always good to plan and prepare before making a video. Imagine where the meeting is going to take place. Think about what you want to achieve in this meeting – what you want the outcome to be. Think about what you want to say – what you want to ask – what you need to know.

Tell me about the room you will be in.
Who is there?
Are they/you sitting or standing?
Describe how each person is looking.
What happens next?
Tell me about the conversation that takes place.
What do you say?
How do you look?

Now it is time to start making the video. Remember you can pause – edit – stop – or delete and start again at any time. It does not matter how many times you pause – edit – stop – or delete and start again. You can keep working on the video until it is just as you want it to be.

*(Guidance note: the hypnotherapist should let the client work on the video for a while and then ask what has been happening in it – some suggestions are presented below)*

How is it going?
What have you done so far?
How is it looking?
How are feeling about it?
What do you still need to do?
Tell me when it is finished.

How were you were feeling as you were making the video?

*(Guidance note: the client's feelings should be explored in detail before proceeding)*

Now I want you to play back the video and watch it. Tell me when you get to the end.

How did you feel as you watched the video?
What are you thinking about the video now?
Tell me what you saw in the video.
How did you look in the video? (*e.g. facial expression; body language; movement*)
How did you look when you were speaking?
How did you look when you were listening to (*insert person/people*)?
What did you say?
What did they say?
How did they react? (*e.g. facial expression; body language; movement*)
Does anything need to be changed/added/deleted?
Do you want to change anything you said – the words or sentences?
Do you want to change how you said what you said? (*e.g. voice - tone; volume; pace of speech; use of emphasis*)
Do you want to say anything else in the video?
Do you want to practise anything else in the video?

> *(Guidance note: if more work does need to be done on the video the hypnotherapist works with the client until they are happy with it)*

Congratulations on creating this video. You have worked hard on this by thinking – planning – preparing for the meeting. The video is ready to be uploaded on to (*insert client's name*)'s Tube. This is very exciting – launching your first (*insert number when more videos are made*) video. Feel that excitement as you upload it now. There it is – well done.

## Option 2: The need to talk/vent

I know sometimes it is hard to talk about certain situations or how you are feeling, when a person or other people are right in front of you. It can be helpful to talk or vent – and it can make you feel so much better. I thought you might like to create a video for (*insert client's name*)'s Tube so that you can tell people about (*insert any of the following as appropriate to the client*):

You
The regrets you have
How the regrets make you feel
Your thoughts
Your feelings
What you do: your behaviours; the ways you cope
How you feel about *(a person)*
How you feel about what happened
How you feel about what you did/did not do
How you feel about what you said/did not say.

You can just sit and talk into your phone and make the video. No-one is going to watch you. You are free to say whatever you want. Let it all out – your thoughts and feelings. So just take some time now – think about what you want to say. Remember it is always good to plan and prepare. I shall be quiet for a short while you gather your thoughts – think about what you want to say.

*(Guidance note: the hypnotherapist should remain quiet for up to two minutes)*

OK. I think it might be helpful to have a rehearsal first before you start recording. So pick up your phone – imagine you are going to record but you won't because this is just a rehearsal. Now talk to your phone. Say what you want to say out loud.

*(Guidance note: the hypnotherapist listens while the client speaks to the phone. Then a discussion should follow. The hypnotherapist can give some feedback after the following general questions have been asked)*

How do you feel about that rehearsal?
Do you want to make any changes before you record the video?

OK are you ready to record? Remember you can pause – edit – stop – or delete and start again at any time It does not matter how many times you pause – edit – stop – or delete and start again. You can keep working on the video until it is just as you want it to be. Start recording and speak out loud now.

*(Guidance note: if the client does pause, edit, stop, delete or start again the hypnotherapist will talk to them about this as and when it happens)*

How did you feel as you were recording what you wanted to say?
Did you say everything you wanted to say?

Now I want you to play back the video and watch it. Tell me when you get to the end.

How did you feel as you watched the video?
What are you thinking about the video now?
Tell me what you saw in the video.
How did you look in the video? (*e.g. facial expression; body language; movement*)
Does anything need to be changed/added/deleted?
Do you want to change anything you said – the words or sentences?
Do you want to change how you said what you said? (*e.g. voice – tone; volume; pace of speech; use of emphasis*)
Do you want to say anything else in the video?

*(Guidance note: if more work does need to be done on the video the hypnotherapist works with the client until they are happy with it)*

Congratulations on creating this video. You have said what you wanted to say. You spoke slowly – clearly – with confidence (*and insert anything else that is appropriate e.g. passion, feeling etc*). The video is ready to be uploaded on to (*insert client's name*)'s Tube. This is very exciting – launching your first (*insert number when more videos are made*) video. Feel that excitement as you upload it now. There it is – well done.

Chapter 32

# I'm sorry

## Introduction

The word "sorry" can just trip off the tongue automatically without giving much thought to it at all. It can be an automatic reaction – a thing to say. When a client, who is working on regrets, needs to make amends for what they have done it is beneficial to spend some time getting them to think about what they are actually sorry about. This is vital in order to prepare and rehearse what the client wants to say if they are planning to meet up with someone in order to say sorry. Just saying sorry is often not enough – some explanation is needed. A hypnotherapist might have to work with a client who has previously (and now regrets):

• Bullied someone
• Abused someone
• Committed a crime
• Left someone e.g. partner/child/family.

I believe it is important for a hypnotherapist to allocate sufficient time with such a client to understand what they are sorry about exactly.

## The script

You have told me that you are sorry about (*insert what has been disclosed previously*). I want you to think about what you are sorry about exactly. It is so easy to say the word "sorry" without really thinking about what you mean. I think it is quite commonplace for people to respond quickly – to say things – without pausing for thought before they open their mouth. How many times has something come out of your mouth and then you thought "I wish I had not said that"? It is so easy to respond to situations without thinking about what you are saying and how people might react to what you have said. You do not think about what you are saying or what you are meaning. It is just an automatic reaction.

The word "sorry" is often said robotically. The use of the single word "sorry" can become a habit. That single word "sorry" can be said without any intonation in

DOI: 10.4324/9781003468325-37

your voice, so it may seem as if you do not really mean it – you are devoid of any feeling. Just think about everyday situations when people say sorry automatically – when accidently bumping into someone in a crowd or on the street – or when a person waiting tables in a restaurant receives a complaint about the food being cold.

Sorry is often said very quickly and there is no further conversation. The person waiting tables in the restaurant may immediately say sorry, pick up the plate and take it back to the kitchen without another word. It is also important to think about body language – what is that telling you? The person cannot wait to get away fast enough rather than talk about what has just happened or been said. Ultimately, the questions that must be asked are:

Does that person actually care?
Are they really sorry?

So now think about the conversation you need to have with (*insert person*).

*(Guidance note: the hypnotherapist needs to probe deeply and work with client in order to plan for the future conversation)*

Do you care?
What do you care about?
Why do you care?
Are you really sorry?
What are you sorry about exactly?
Are you sorry about what you said/did not say?
Are you sorry about what you did/did not do?
What do want to say to *(insert person)*?

Let's plan that now – what you are going to say exactly.

*(Guidance note: the hypnotherapist can then get the client to plan and rehearse. It can be useful to use this script in conjunction with the script in Chapter 29 "The meeting room")*

# Part VI

# Releasing

# Chapter 33

# The drainage system

## Introduction

This script uses the imagery of water and the drainage system to release the regrets. The flowing water takes the regrets away by travelling through drains, water pipes, sewers and eventually into the sea and out to the ocean. The hypnotherapist can choose to reinsert the concept of travelling along the road of regrets when using this script.

## The script

All around the country local water companies are repairing and replacing old water pipes. Have you ever thought about how many water pipes there might be under the roads? Some of the pipes are very old and leak, so now there is so much work going on to replace old pipes and make the drainage system more efficient. Now I wonder if you have ever thought about how many drains there might be. Drains can lead from houses, shops and all kinds of buildings – they are a place where waste accumulates and then connects to the main water pipes and sewers underneath the roads. Taking away the things we do not need or we do not want anymore. Just start to let your mind flow – flow like water – and think about the drains – the water pipes – and the sewers. Just let your mind flow and flow and flow – just like water – flow and flow and flow. See all those – drains – water pipes – and sewers – carrying away all that waste.

Think about the waste you have accumulated. Waste can take many forms – waste can be many things. Waste is something that is no longer useful – it has served its purpose. Waste can form at the end of a process, which has been completed. Waste is something you do not need anymore. Waste is something you do not want anymore. You have worked on your regrets – they have served their purpose – now they are something you do not need anymore. They are something you do not want anymore. They are waste and they need to be thrown away.

So imagine you are standing outside a house – any house – it does not matter where it is. I want you to find a drain – a drain you would like to use to get rid of your waste. It might be on a driveway – in a garden – at the side of a patio – or in

DOI: 10.4324/9781003468325-39

a back yard. It might be one of those that has a manhole cover on the top of the drain. Or maybe you will find a drain on the road – one of those that has a grid on the top of it and you can see right down. Have a wander around – explore around the outside of the house – explore the road. Tell me when you have found the drain you want to use. Drains go down very, very deep. Down and down and down – very, very deep.

*(Guidance note: if the client does see a drain with a manhole cover it will be necessary to get the client to remove the cover before proceeding)*

Describe the drain to me.
How far down can you see?
Tell me what you can see exactly.
Now think about the regrets you have been working through.

*(Guidance note: some hypnotherapists may want to remind the client of the work that has been undertaken and if a regrets list has been completed this can be used as a summary reminder/prompt)*

Now it is time to throw your regrets – the waste – into the drain. Start to do that now. Tell me what you are throwing down the drain.

*(Guidance note: the hypnotherapist should keep talking with the client as each regret is thrown down the drain and repeat: "Drains go down very, very deep. Down and down and down – very, very deep")*

How are you feeling as you are throwing the regrets – the waste – away?

Now all the regrets are in the drain. The regrets are waste – you no longer have any need for them. You no longer want them in your life. They have served their purpose. I want you to think about the fact that drains go down very, very deep. Down and down and down – very, very deep. Imagine your regrets falling down and down the drain – and plummeting into a pipe – a water pipe. Water is flowing through the pipe and it is going to take the regrets into the sewers. See the regrets in the water pipe – they start to move forward – they are going into the sewers. I wonder if you can smell anything. You see the regrets being carried forward by the water. The water is moving slowly at first but then it gathers momentum and it travels at a faster pace – the water is gaining speed. Watch the regrets – the waste – being carried away. Travelling faster and faster along the water pipe.

If some bits of waste get stuck, the water will come along and push them along. The regrets are not sticking to anything. The water is washing them away. They cannot stick – they have to keep travelling – moving away.

Soon that water pipe will meet another water pipe and another water pipe. The drainage system is like a map. In some places the pipes come together – in other places they part ways and go in different directions. Ultimately, the drainage system will flush out the waste into the sea. Keep watching the regrets – the waste – travelling along the water pipes – travelling through the drainage system – going further away – further and further away. The water keeps washing them away. Keep watching and feel them rushing away.

The waste is getting nearer to the sea now. Imagine the sea – the strong, powerful, deep sea. It is not far away. The waste will be flushed into the sea and then the sea will take it out to the ocean. The waste is so near the exit of the pipe now. The water is pushing hard. There will be one last push and whoosh the waste is pushed into the sea. Now watch the sea carry the waste out towards the ocean. The waste is carried away. The waste has been disposed of – gone forever.

Chapter 34

# Cliff edge

## Introduction

This is a good script to use when most of the work with regrets has been done. It definitely should not be used for anyone who has a fear of heights. The script acknowledges that the client has been on a hard, steep climb working through their regrets and the cliff edge is now a place to throw away the regrets into the sea. Before using the script, if more than one regret has been worked on then the hypnotherapist should have written down a list of the regrets which have been addressed in previous sessions (Appendix 5.2 can be used for this purpose). In the script I have referred to regrets because in my experience it is usual for a client to have more than one regret which they need to work on. However, if only one regret has been worked on then the single use of the word should be used.

## The script

Just imagine it is a day at the beginning of spring. Spring is a time of hope – a time when things are born – come alive – grow. It is a time for fresh starts – new beginnings. I want you to imagine that you are outside somewhere. The air feels warm on your face and hands. You look up to the sky and you can see the sun. Feel the warmth coming down from the sun – warming the earth. You are going to take a walk. A gentle walk – you do not have to hurry – there is no rush at all. It is good to take time for yourself. I want you to enjoy the walk. Relax. So just start walking forwards.

As you are walking breathe in slowly and deeply – and then breathe out very gently. That's right. You know how to do this. You know breathing helps you relax. So again – breathe in slowly and deeply – and then breathe out very gently. Slowly – deeply – and then very gently. Good – keep walking forward – keep breathing – slowly – deeply – and then very gently. That's right. Slowly – deeply – and then very gently.

As you walk forward you become aware that the path you are following is going upwards. Just walk slowly – you do not have to hurry. You can cope with the path going upwards. Look around as you walk. Take some more deep breaths. You may

DOI: 10.4324/9781003468325-40

become aware of smelling or tasting salt – salt from the sea. I wonder if you can hear the sound of the sea. Keep climbing the pathway upwards.

As you are walking and relaxing at your own pace – I want you to start thinking about the regrets we have been talking about in our sessions. You have been doing so well opening up – identifying your regrets – talking about them – working through them. Think about your regrets as you keep walking upwards. If the pathway feels as though it is getting steeper slow down a bit – take some more deep breaths – and take things in your stride. You know that you can. There is no need to rush. You can cope with the pathway going upwards. Keep thinking about the regrets you have had. Climbing up this pathway may remind you of how hard it is sometimes to deal with regrets – acknowledging what has happened or not happened – but you have done it – worked through your regrets – and now you are going to climb to the top of this pathway.

You are going up and up. Keep going. The pathway is becoming even steeper now. You notice on either side of the pathway that there is some grass – some rocks – and then you notice some bits of sand. You realise you are climbing a cliff. The calf muscles in your legs may be aching – but you keep going – you do not give up. You can get to the top of the cliff – the view at the top will be worth the effort you are putting in. Keep going. Up – and up – and up. Keep going.

You are nearly there now. Imagine seeing the sea – hearing the waves – seeing the seagulls flying high in the sky. Almost there now – just a little bit further. Up and up – nearly at the top now. Just a little bit further. It is very steep but you are doing so well – you are almost there now. *1, 2,* and *3* and you are there. The ground flattens out. Take a really deep breath – in and out. Stop – rest – and take another really deep breath – in and out. Let your breathing slow down. Prepare yourself to look at the beautiful view. Breathe in slowly and deeply – and then breathe out very gently. And again – breathe in slowly and deeply – and then breathe out very gently. Slowly – deeply – and then very gently.

Look out towards the sea. Across the flat ground you can see the cliff edge. Look up and you see the beautiful blue sky – the warm, bright sun – and the seagulls flying high in the sky. Listen for the waves of the sea. Now you are ready to walk to the edge of the cliff. It is time. Walk forward towards the edge – go as close to the edge as you can – and then stop. Look straight in front of you – what do you see? Now look down – what do you see?

The sea is very deep and it is a really good place to get rid of things. You can throw things away and the current will take those things away – never to be seen again. So I want you to think about the regrets you have worked on. Think about each individual one – name each one.

*(Guidance note: the hypnotherapist should encourage the client to name each regret out loud. The hypnotherapist will check whether the regrets named are on the list which has been prepared. If the client mentions a regret which has not been discussed previously, then the hypnotherapist needs to get more information about this before proceeding)*

Now it is time to get rid of each individual regret you have worked through. One by one you are going to throw a regret into the sea. Which one will you throw first? When you are ready throw the regret – *1, 2,* and *3.* Watch it fly through the air. See it descend into the sea. Watch the ripples it causes. See it disappear – deep into the sea – down and down and down. Sinking – sinking and sinking. Down and down and down. Being pulled out to sea – far, far away – never to return.

What did you feel when you threw (*regret*)?
How do you feel now?

It is time to get rid of the next regret. Which one will it be? When you are ready throw the regret – *1, 2,* and *3.* Watch it fly through the air. See it descend into the sea. Watch the ripples it causes. See it disappear – deep into the sea – down and down and down. Sinking – sinking and sinking. Down and down and down. Being pulled out to sea – far, far away – never to return.

> *(Guidance note: the client will continue to throw away each individual regret and the hypnotherapist will encourage discussion about how this feels)*

Well done. You have thrown away all your regrets. They are gone forever. It is very natural to have regrets – some are harder to face than others. You have faced them and you have worked through them. You have learnt from them and today you have released them. Now you can plan for the future – but that can wait for another day. It is time to relax now. Come back from the cliff edge. Find yourself a comfortable spot somewhere on the flat part of the cliff. Sit down or lie down – make yourself comfortable – focus on your breathing. Breathe in slowly and deeply – and then breathe out very gently. Slowly – deeply – and then very gently.

Listen to the sounds around you. Breathe in slowly and deeply – and then breathe out very gently. Slowly – deeply – and then very gently. Feel the warmth of the sun on your face. Breathe in slowly and deeply – and then breathe out very gently. Slowly – deeply – and then very gently.

That's right – just relax.

# Chapter 35

# Ice cubes melting

## Introduction

The main purpose of this script is to melt away some of the common negative feelings which are experienced by a client who is having regrets. When working on regrets I have often heard clients describe themselves as being:

- Cold
- Hardened
- Bitter
- Detached
- Isolated
- Bad tempered
- Furious
- Angry.

In the script, ice cubes and a hot tub are used to melt away negative feelings the client has and acknowledge that extreme temperatures can be experienced.

## The script

You are standing still in a car park when you see the entrance to a supermarket in front of you. You are aware of people going into the supermarket – adults – children – babies in buggies. Other people are coming out either pushing trolleys or carrying bags. You are going to enter the supermarket very shortly. You know what you need to find – bags of ice cubes. You will need a trolley so look around and find one before you go into the supermarket. Hold the handle of the trolley firmly. The trolley has sturdy wheels and will lead you in the right direction. You know what you need to do. You know the time is right. So start walking with the trolley towards the entrance of the supermarket. Now go into the supermarket.

It is very busy. There are lots of people in the supermarket. Some people are in a rush; others are sauntering around taking their time. You need to find the frozen food section – where the bags of ice cubes will be stored in a freezer. So start

DOI: 10.4324/9781003468325-41

walking up and down the aisles. No need to rush. Walk down the various aisles and maybe you will see all different types of food – vegetables – fruit – meats – fish – cheese – packets of cereals – biscuits – all sorts of tins – dairy products – milk – cream – yoghurt. There will be drinks too and lots of other things – stationery – books – toys – household items – clothes. Find your way to the frozen food section. As you get nearer you feel the air around you becoming colder. You know you are getting nearer. The air around you is getting colder and colder. You see the freezers and walk towards them. Now walk around and find the freezer which has the bags of ice cubes.

Just stand and look at the bags of ice cubes. There are so many of them. Feel the coldness coming out of the freezer. You feel the coldness on your face – on your hands. The ice cubes are very, very cold – they are ice cold. Water has been frozen to make them into solid cubes of ice. Put one of your hands into the freezer and just rest the palm of your hand on one bag of ice cubes. Feel the cold. Keep your hand there. The bag of ice cubes feels very solid – there is no movement inside the bag. Some of the ice cubes have stuck together – they have become a solid mass. Even though the bag is freezing cold it may feel as though your hand is burning – the ice is burning your hand. Feel the sharpness of pain. Now take your hand off the bag of ice cubes. Feel the stinging in the palm of your hand, which may linger for a while.

The bag of ice cubes is like some of the feelings you have been experiencing. Feelings can be at opposite ends of the temperature gauge. Sometimes very cold – or freezing – sometimes very hot – almost burning. If a person cuts off their feelings they do not have to feel anything at all. It seems easier to cope that way – you do not have to feel any pain or anything at all. A person can harden up – cut themselves off – they become very isolated – they feel alone – and out in the cold. That can bring anger forward, which is at the other end of the temperature gauge. The anger rages and makes the person feel as though they are burning up – maybe out of control. A person can be cold and hot at the same time. The feelings become muddled and confusing.

You have experienced different feelings. You have been working through your feelings. You have talked about feeling (*insert feelings discussed in previous sessions*). Is there anything else you have been feeling?

*(Guidance note: if the client does bring forward other feelings the hypnotherapist should allow time to discuss these thoroughly before working further with the bags of ice cubes)*

Now it is time to melt all those feelings away. So look at the bags of ice cubes in the freezer. Decide how many bags you need. Then take the bags out of the freezer and place them in the trolley. As you pick up the bags of ice cubes feel the coldness again and the burning sensations in your hands. Wheel the trolley to the check out and pay for the bags of ice cubes. Now walk out of the supermarket. Push the trolley forward. The trolley is going to take you to another place – a place which is much warmer. So keep pushing the trolley. The trolley knows the way – the right way to go to find a warmer place. Keep pushing the trolley. Soon you will see a very big hot tub in the distance. You feel the air getting warmer. You notice some water on the outside of the bags of ice cubes. Keep pushing the trolley. It is getting warmer and warmer.

Now you see the very big hot tub clearly – it is right in front of you. It is full of boiling hot water – you see the steam rising up from the hot tub. Take the bags of ice cubes out of the trolley and place them on the floor. Place both your hands on the bags of ice cubes. They are still freezing cold but not as cold as they were before. They have started to defrost on the journey to the hot tub. Some of the ice cubes which had stuck together have started to separate. They are not so hard. There is movement – some flexibility within the bags. Now it is time to melt the ice cubes. Melt away the coldness – hardness – the burning sensation. So you need to open the bags and then you are going to pour the ice cubes into the hot tub. Tell me when you are ready to do this. Ready to get rid of the feelings you do not need anymore.

Lean over the side of the hot tub – see the boiling water – feel the steam rising up onto your face. Now pour the ice cubes into the boiling hot water and watch them melt. See the ice cubes melting away – getting smaller and smaller. Watch the ice cubes melting – melting – melting away until they are no more. Keep watching until they have melted completely into the boiling water. The boiling water is cooling down as the ice cubes are melting away. The water is becoming cooler – it is getting down to just the right temperature – just the right temperature for you. Tell me when all the ice cubes have melted away.

So now it is time for you to climb into the hot tub and sit down. It is time to relax and feel good. The water is just the right temperature for you. You feel relaxed – you feel good – you feel comfortable. What else are you feeling?

*(Guidance note: the hypnotherapist should wait for a response and have some discussion about how the client is feeling. It is helpful for the client to relax in the hot tub for a while before proceeding further)*

Chapter 36

# Bubble machine

## Introduction

This script is another script which can be used when the client has worked through their regrets and they are ready to release the regrets. Using a bubble machine facilitates this process by blowing out bubbles, some of which contain the client's regrets. When all the regrets have floated away the client gets into their own bubble and floats into their future.

## The script

Take some deep breaths in and out. I want you to get a lot of air into your lungs. Feel the power within your lungs as you breathe in and fill your lungs with air – and then breathe out. Keep taking really deep breaths – in and out – keep going. As you breathe in feel the clean air filling your lungs. Feel your lungs expanding. Feel the strength and power in your lungs. As you breathe out, feel the air expelling from your lungs slowly. Continue to breathe really deeply – in and out. Feel the strength and power in your lungs. Your lungs are expanding – gaining in strength – so when you need to blow out hard you will be able to do so with confidence. Keep taking really deep breaths.

Now that you feel energised I want you to imagine that you are outside. You see a garden – a beautiful garden – full of trees – bushes – flowers – and so much more. Take another deep breath in and see if you can smell anything from the garden – and then breathe out. Look up into the beautiful clear blue sky – there are no clouds to be seen anywhere. You feel a very gentle breeze but it is hardly noticeable at all. Walk into the garden and have a look around. You see a shed in the garden, which houses many different things. You are going to go into the shed and look for a bubble machine – a small machine that can make bubbles. Look for the bubble machine – it will be somewhere in the shed. Tell me when you have found it. Go back into the garden and decide where you would like to place the bubble machine. You are going to need some bubble solution to put in the machine. Go back into the shed and find a big bottle of bubble solution. Tell me when you have found it.

DOI: 10.4324/9781003468325-42

Look at the bubble machine and find the place where you can put in the bubble solution. Open the bottle of bubble solution and fill the machine right up – so it can make lots and lots of bubbles. Somewhere on the bubble machine there will be a button to push – this will make the bubble machine blow bubbles out. It is always lovely to watch bubbles float into the air – so light and free to travel wherever they want to go. Today the bubble machine has a particular job to do. It will produce bubbles that contain your regrets. The regrets you have been working through. It is now time for the regrets to be blown away. They need to be released into the air – to be blown away – far, far, away – never to be seen again.

So on the count of *3*, I want you to push the button on the machine and watch for the bubbles to appear. *1, 2*, and *3* – push the button and wait for the bubbles to start coming out of the bubble machine. See one bubble – then another – more bubbles start appearing. Some are small – some are medium-sized – others are really big. Some bubbles which burst out of the bubble machine are a long, thin shape and then they form into a round bubble. Watch the bubbles – see through the bubbles. I wonder if you can see any colours in the walls of the bubbles. Keep watching the bubbles on their journey. Watch the bubbles – travelling in all directions – so light – so free. Travelling upwards – to the right – to the left – up and up and up they float towards the sky. So light – so free. Travelling in all directions. Travelling upwards – to the right – to the left – up and up and up they float. So light – so free. Travelling in all directions. All the bubbles are travelling at their own speed. Some move very quickly – others go at a more leisurely pace – but they all keep moving – they do not stop.

Now some of the bubbles are carrying your regrets. Look for the bubbles which are carrying your regrets. Start to see your regrets in some of the bubbles. Which regrets do you see?

*(Guidance note: the hypnotherapist should encourage discussion about the bubbles, which are carrying regrets, i.e. which regrets are being seen by the client)*

Now it is time to say goodbye to the regrets. You no longer need them. Thank them for being there – for serving a purpose – but now you need to let them go. It is time for you to continue your life without them. Feel the lightness growing within you as you watch the bubbles travelling in all directions – upwards – to the right – to the left. Upwards they go – higher and higher – feeling lighter and lighter. Watch the bubbles go in all directions – upwards and upwards. Upwards they go – higher and higher – feeling lighter and lighter. Say goodbye to the regrets – watch them float away – watch them float out of sight.

Now you need to check whether any more regrets need to be released or whether you can just enjoy watching the bubbles travel in all directions.

*(Guidance note: sometimes all the regrets will be identified in the first set of bubbles which comes out of the machine. In other cases, the client needs to push*

*the button on the bubble machine more than once and work through the regrets in the different groups of bubbles which appear. When this happens the client keeps pushing the button on the bubble machine until the bubble solution runs out)*

Push the button on the bubble machine again. More bubbles come out. The bubbles are all different sizes. Watch the bubbles – see through the bubbles. I wonder if you can see any colours in the walls of the bubbles. Keep watching the bubbles on their journey. Watch the bubbles – travelling in all directions – so light – so free. Travelling upwards – to the right – to the left – up and up and up they float towards the sky. So light – so free. Travelling in all directions. Travelling upwards – to the right – to the left – up and up and up they float. So light – so free. Travelling in all directions. Look at these bubbles and see if any of them are carrying any more regrets.

*(Guidance note: If more regrets appear repeat as follows)*

Now it is time to say goodbye to the regrets. You no longer need them. Thank them for being there – for serving a purpose – but now you need to let them go. It is time for you to continue your life without them. Feel the lightness growing within you as you watch the bubbles travelling in all directions – upwards – to the right – to the left. Upwards they go – higher and higher – feeling lighter and lighter. Watch the bubbles go in all directions – upwards and upwards. Upwards they go – higher and higher – feeling lighter and lighter. Say goodbye to the regrets – watch them float away – watch them float out of sight.

*(Guidance note: When all the regrets have floated away – continue)*

Keep watching until all the bubbles have disappeared. There are no bubbles to be seen anywhere in the garden or in the air – or high in the sky. All the bubbles have gone – gone completely. Now there is just one more thing that needs to happen. First of all, top up the bubble machine with some bubble solution. On the count of 3 – push the button on the bubble machine again – *1, 2, and 3*. Watch one bubble start to come out of the bubble machine. Look at the one bubble as it is pushed out of the machine. It looks long and thin. It starts to get longer – then it gets wider. You can see it evolving into a bubble shape – a round bubble. The bubble is now formed – a perfect circle.

Focus your attention on the one bubble as it hovers by the bubble machine. As you watch the bubble it starts to get bigger and bigger and bigger. Watch how large it grows – wait until it is large enough for you to walk into it. Bigger and bigger and bigger. Now it is big enough for you to walk into the bubble. Step into the bubble now and feel a shift in how you feel. You feel safe – protected. You also feel excited – wanting to float in the bubble – you can go anywhere you want to go – you can go in whichever direction you want to travel – you can even travel in more than one direction.

So on the count of *3* – start your journey in the bubble – float with the bubble – *1, 2,* and *3.* The bubble starts floating – it such a lovely feeling. You feel safe in the bubble. You can just let the bubble float freely or you can tell the bubble which way you want it to go. It is completely up to you – it is your decision. Think about what you want to do now that you have said goodbye to your regrets. They have gone forever. Now is the time to plan for the future. You do not have to rush – just take your time – you have plenty of time to float into your future.

Enjoy being inside the bubble as it continues to float. It feels light inside the bubble – you feel light within you. Up and up and up you float. Higher and higher into the beautiful clear blue sky. Keep going higher and as you do so, look down through the bubble and see what you want for your future.

Chapter 37

# Army of ants

## Introduction

This script uses a colony of ants to take away the client's regrets. It embeds the idea of getting a job done systematically – having a plan and a strategy. There is also an emphasis on feeling upright, steady and secure.

## The script

You are standing on a patio. The patio is laid with flat, smooth paving stones which give you a feeling of being upright, steady and secure. Look around for a chair and then sit down on it. You are going to go into trance – a deep trance state. You are feeling relaxed but also you recognise other feelings deep within you – motivation – and determination. Going deeper and deeper into a deep trance state now – such a lovely feeling – feeling relaxed – completely relaxed.

Look at the patio. Look at the paving stones. Look around the patio. Look into every corner of the patio. I wonder what you are seeing. Maybe some plant pots – plants – ornaments – some furniture. Become aware of your surroundings. The fresh, clean air around you. The sky above you. The sun shining down bringing gentle warmth onto the patio. You sense movement. Birds flying in the sky. Maybe some butterflies – bees – wasps – insects. Sense the gentle movement around you – really sense it. You then become aware of some quicker movement – busy movement – giving you a sense there is some urgency. You look down and you see an ant running across the patio. You watch the ant and as you do so you see another ant running in the opposite direction. Then you see another one. It looks like this one is carrying a piece of bread. Then the ant scuttles away and disappears.

As you watch more closely you see more and more ants appearing on the patio. They run across the patio in all different directions – from one side to the other – from top to bottom – diagonally. Some of the ants go round in circles – round and round and round. They look so busy. It may look chaotic but the ants are actually working together systematically. They know exactly what they doing and each ant knows its role in this colony of ants. The colony of ants is like an army. It has a plan to get a job done. It has a strategy – how the job will get completed successfully.

DOI: 10.4324/9781003468325-43

The ants have knowledge and skills to implement the plan and they will put the plan into action. They will succeed and get the job done quickly and efficiently.

You have been working to a plan. The plan has been to work through your regrets, release them and go forward to live your life without regrets. Today it is time to move and release the regrets and the army of ants will help you do this. They are willing and able – just like you are willing and able to let the regrets go. It is going to be a smooth and quick operation.

Now watch as more ants come onto the patio. These ants are carrying your regrets. Notice how the ants work in small groups to carry the regrets. The ants which have already been on the patio for a while are now gathering together – they are manoeuvring themselves into lines. The new ants that are bringing your regrets onto the patio are placing the regrets on the backs of the ants that are standing in lines. Watch the operation carefully. The ants are working systematically. They know exactly what they have to do – where to place the regrets so they are in a secure position – they will not fall off the backs of the ants onto the patio. The army of ants are going to carry the regrets off the patio. Keep watching the operation. The ants are busy working to a plan. They know exactly what they have to do. They know how this operation will work – they know the correct manoeuvres to use in order to carry things away. Keep watching as the ants put all the regrets on top of the army of ants.

Look at more lines of ants forming. See how the ants get into position – how they are preparing themselves to get the job done. Their movements slow down as they all come together. All the ants become still. Together they are a very strong force. They have the strength to move the regrets and take them off the patio – away from you. You are done with the regrets. They have served their purpose. You have no need of them anymore. You do not need to see the regrets anymore. Sense the stillness. Sense the strength of the army. Sense the readiness – readiness to move forward. Sense the anticipation – anticipation to get the job done.

Suddenly the front line of the army starts to move. The other lines then start to move. They move forward quickly – there is no hesitation. The ants are upright – steady – and keep the regrets securely on their backs. They are capable of carrying the regrets away quickly – there is no hesitation. The ants are upright – steady – and keep the regrets securely on their backs. Watch as the ants move along the patio – taking the regrets away from you. You are done with the regrets. You do not need to see the regrets anymore. Watch the lines of ants going away from you. The regrets are being carried away. Feel the relief – the lightness growing inside you. Let the regrets go with the army of ants – let the regrets go forever. Keep watching as the ants take the regrets off the patio and go into the distance – far away. Keep watching the army – the movement – into the distance – far away. Feel the relief – the lightness growing inside you. Keep watching until all the lines of ants have disappeared. All the regrets have gone.

Just relax for a while longer. Enjoy relaxing in the chair on the patio. Look at the flat, smooth paving stones. You can now pave your way into the future – feeling upright – steady – and secure.

# Chapter 38

# Flying with the birds

## Introduction

In Part IV of the book, which is concerned with working through emotions, several scripts deal with feelings of being stuck or trapped. The script in this chapter returns to these two feelings and aims to work on leaving the situation which has created the feeling of being stuck or trapped by flying away with birds and then experiencing freedom. It is a script clients often want to return to in order to feel free; and consequently, the script can be used for relaxation purposes.

In the script I have used the words stuck/trapped. It may be that the client uses different terminology which implies being stuck or trapped. Children in particular may have used very different words to describe these feelings. The hypnotherapist can adapt the script to include words that are meaningful to the client. The script works well for both children and adults. Using the client's own language is best practice in order to work in a person-centred way.

## The script

You have told me about how you have felt stuck/trapped (*or use any particular word the client has used*). It is now time to work on getting rid of that feeling. I want you to go back to a time when you felt stuck/trapped (*or insert another word*). Imagine the situation. Remember the place where you were. Remember what was happening. Remember how you were feeling. Experience that feeling again. I know this may feel uncomfortable but try to stay with it. I shall be quiet for a short time while you start to remember and experience that situation and experience that feeling.

*(Guidance note: the hypnotherapist should stay quiet for between 30 seconds and a full minute; and then continue with the following questions to get more information about the client's feeling of being stuck/trapped)*

Tell me where you are.
Is anyone else there?

DOI: 10.4324/9781003468325-44

What is happening?
Describe to me how you are feeling.
What happens next?

*(Guidance note: if the client is describing a situation which is taking place inside use the following paragraph to get them outside before proceeding)*

### If the client is inside

You are now going to leave this feeling behind. I know it may feel as though you cannot move but you can and you will move. You are going to go outside in order to move away. You can and you will move. On the count of *3* – start to walk – *1*, *2*, and *3*. Walk out of that situation. Keep walking until you find yourself outside and keep walking until you are a long way from that situation.

### If the client is already outside

You are now going to leave this feeling behind. I know it may feel as though you cannot move but you can and you will move. You are going to move away. You can and you will move. On the count of *3* – start to walk – *1*, *2*, and *3*. Walk out of that situation. Keep walking until you are a long way from that situation.

### Continue

It is a warm, bright day. Look up to the sky. You can see it is blue and there are some little white clouds scattered about. Keep watching the sky. You see some birds flying about. Keep watching – some more birds might fly into view. The birds are circling in the sky. See how graceful they are. Flying easily through the sky – through the clouds. They look so free – able to go anywhere they want to go. Keep watching the birds – they are gathering together. Flying round and round.

You suddenly notice that the birds are flying down towards the ground. They are coming towards you. The birds are getting nearer and nearer now – closer and closer. They have almost reached you. Then they are there. They tug at your clothing in a friendly, safe way. Then you realise they are using their beaks to lift you off the ground. Your feet are off the ground. You feel safe amongst the birds that are surrounding you. They are lifting you higher and higher – and as they do so you realise that you no longer have any feeling of being stuck/trapped. The birds are lifting you higher and higher. You are free. You have left that feeling of being stuck/trapped on the ground. You feel free – free to go wherever you want to go. Do whatever you want to do.

The birds keep taking you higher and higher. Enjoy this experience. Look all around you – up into the sky – around you – and down to the ground. You are safe and free. You are going to experience new feelings as you travel up and up through the sky. Look around you.

Tell me what you can see.
How are you feeling?

Look down at the ground – see what you have left behind. You are no longer feeling stuck/trapped.

Where do you want to go now?
What do you want to do in the future?
Where do you want to go in the future?

The birds will always be there for you. You can talk to them. You can ask them questions. You can fly with them just for fun or they will always be there to help you get away from situations you do not want to be in. Remember you can talk to them. You can ask them questions. They will pick you up and fly with you – go anywhere you want to go. You can fly with the birds anytime you want – just look to the sky and watch for the birds.

# Chapter 39

# Dusting and hoovering up

## Introduction

Regrets and the thoughts, feelings and behaviours associated with them, can become embedded within the subconscious mind. This can result in people having repetitive thoughts and feelings, so the way a person responds to having regrets becomes a habit. In the script the client will imagine dusting dust particles away (the thoughts and feelings) and hoovering up the dirt (the regrets), which are deeply embedded in the carpet's deep pile.

## The script

I wonder how much you think about dust, dust particles and actual dirt. I want you to think about those things now. Dust can be irritating. It flies about – it can get up your nose – it can make you sneeze and it can make you feel itchy. Dust particles can be so small it is hard to see them and therefore hard to get rid of them. You can be chasing them for a long time. Even when you have dusted them away, they can fly back and land somewhere else. Dusting can be a very frustrating task. Actual dirt can take many forms – it can be heavy – light – small – large – sticky – mucky – and sometimes smelly. Like dust and dust particles, real dirt can be hard to dispose of – especially if it becomes ground in somewhere.

Imagine now that you are going to do some dusting. You are in a room somewhere and you have a duster in your hand. You may see a door – a window or maybe more than one window – and there will be some furniture around you. Tell me what you are seeing.

Now look around – see if you can see dust on any of the surfaces. If you do see some dust, start dusting – get rid of the dust – get rid of the dust particles. Some of them may fly away into the air and try to return. Keep dusting. You know you can get rid of the dust. The dust particles are like some of the thoughts and feelings you have been experiencing and talking about. They may seem very light and not too much of a problem, but they keep coming back and that can be very irritating. So as you continue to dust, think about some of the thoughts and feelings you have been experiencing.

DOI: 10.4324/9781003468325-45

Look hard into the dust and dust particles as you keep dusting. I wonder how they make you feel – especially when they keep coming back. You know that if you keep dusting you can get rid of the dust particles forever – they will never return. So keep dusting hard – get rid of those particles. Keep dusting hard. Make sure the surfaces you are dusting are left clean and shiny. The surfaces will be clean and shiny – ready for other things to be placed on them – they will not be dusty any-more. New things can replace the dust.

Now dust and dust particles may be irritating but you can get rid of them by dusting, because they are small and light. Real dirt can be heavy and difficult to shift, but it can be done. Look at the carpet on the floor. What colour is the carpet? This carpet is good quality – the pile is deep – it is thick and hard wearing. Over time things have dropped onto the carpet and if they are not cleared up at the time, they can become trodden into the pile. As people walk over the carpet the dirt can sink down – sink down and down – further into the carpet. Look now at the deep pile – touch the pile – feel the texture – thick – good quality. Look and feel. Maybe you feel some dirt in the carpet. Rub your hand along the carpet. I wonder if it is sticky – gritty – or hard – very hard. I wonder how the carpet feels to you. Dirt can be hard to shift but it can be done. You can and you will shift the dirt.

Look deep into the carpet. Look at the pile. Imagine how deep it is – how far it goes down. Now think about the regrets you have – the regrets which have been coming into your mind – the regrets that keep returning – the regrets that have been affecting your life – affecting your thoughts – affecting your feelings – and affecting your behaviours. Imagine those regrets now being in the pile of the carpet. See them embedded deep down in the carpet. Now it is time to get them out of the carpet.

Somewhere in the room there will be a hoover. It will be a very powerful hoover – full of suction. When you find the hoover, plug it into a socket – and then switch it on. Listen to the sound of the hoover – it is loud and powerful. You know that the hoover has the power to suck out all the dirt in the carpet. Think about that power and strength. On the count of *3* you are going to start hoovering. *1, 2* and *3* – start hoovering now. The hoover starts sucking up the dirt.

Push the hoover forwards and backwards – forwards and backwards. Feel the strength of the hoover as you push forwards and backwards. It is gripping the carpet. Feel the power of the hoover's suction. Imagine your regrets – the regrets which have been coming into your mind – the regrets that keep returning – the regrets that have been affecting your life – your thoughts – your feelings – and your behaviours. See your regrets embedded deep down in the pile of the carpet. Watch carefully as the regrets start to loosen. They are no longer stuck in the pile of the carpet. They are becoming looser and looser. They are coming up from the bottom of the pile – up – up and up. Looser and looser. They are being sucked up and out – up and out. They are no longer stuck – they are no longer embedded in the pile of the carpet. They are being sucked up and out – up and out.

The dirt in the carpet is being shifted – sucked up and out – up and out. All the dirt is coming loose – it is coming to the surface – and it will be sucked into the hoover – it cannot escape. The hoover is powerful. The hoover can do a good, thorough job in getting rid of the dirt. Watch the dirt coming up and out of the carpet – into the hoover – and into the hoover bag.

Keep pushing the hoover forwards and backwards – forwards and backwards. Feel the power of the hoover – feel its suction – see the dirt coming up and out – up and out. Look at the carpet – look at the colour of the carpet – it is becoming lighter and lighter – cleaner and cleaner. The carpet is getting a thorough, deep clean. The dirt is going into the hoover – never to escape. The carpet is getting cleaner and cleaner – lighter and lighter. Keep pushing the hoover forwards and backwards until you know there is no more dirt to come out of the carpet. Tell me when you have finished hoovering. Good job. Now you need to empty the hoover bag – empty it of all the dirt. So do that now – take the hoover bag outside and empty the dirt into a dustbin.

The carpet looks fresh and clean. The colour of the carpet is lighter – lighter and lighter. All the dirt has been lifted and it has gone. The final job is to make the carpet ready for the future – so that it will last for years and years as people come and go. So to make it ready for the future you need to shampoo the carpet. The hoover is a machine that can double up as a carpet cleaner. It has a tank in it. You need to find some carpet cleaner and fill up the tank with it. Now shampoo the carpet – make it really clean. Like before, push the hoover forwards and backwards – forwards and backwards. Shampoo the carpet thoroughly – make it fresh and clean – it starts to smell fresh and clean. Push the hoover forwards and backwards – forwards and backwards. Keep shampooing until it is really clean – fresh and clean. Now it is ready to last for years.

# Chapter 40

# Let's have a declutter

## Introduction

Some clients find it very hard to let go of their regrets or rather the repetitive thoughts or feelings that accompany them. The main objective of this script is to help the client to get rid of those thoughts, feelings and behaviours by decluttering a garden shed. The script also focuses on tidying up and organising the future. I have found that this script will often need to be used over two sessions; or even three sessions when there is a lot of decluttering to be done.

## The script

I wonder if you think about people having a declutter you might imagine people clearing out their houses. Well that is a form of decluttering but it can go far beyond that. Decluttering can be very good for you in lots of different ways, if you take it further than just getting rid of physical things – like objects or possessions. It is good to get rid of physical things that take up too much space or maybe hold bad rather than good memories for you. It is equally good to declutter the body and mind of other things too. Decluttering is about removing unnecessary items – things you do not need anymore – and that can include people. Let's do that now. Let's have a declutter of what has been bothering you. Let's have a declutter of your regrets and the things associated with those regrets – thoughts and feelings – and behaviours.

I want you to imagine that you are in a garden. It is a very long, narrow garden. Start walking down the garden – keep walking until you find a shed. Tell me when you find it. Sheds are usually full of things – often some useful things – but also things that are no longer useful or are no longer needed. Sometimes a lot of rubbish accumulates over time in a shed. You need to sort out this shed today – you need to have a declutter. To help you do this, you will see that near the shed there is a very large skip – a place where you can deposit all the stuff that is no longer useful to you and stuff you no longer need.

From the outside, the shed probably looks like an ordinary garden shed. I can tell you that this is a very different type of shed on the inside. Once you step into

DOI: 10.4324/9781003468325-46

it, it will feel like you have entered a cave – because the inside of the shed will feel huge. There will be lots of little spaces and hiding places. So now on the count of *3* open the garden shed door and go in: *1, 2* and *3* – in you go. Look at the huge area you find yourself in – it is full of stuff.

Look around the inside of the shed – look at the floor – the ceiling – the walls. Have a walk around. You may see all sorts of things – maybe tables – chairs – shelves – cupboards – drawers – bookcases – dressers – wardrobes – chests of drawers – chests – boxes. Inside the shed feels so huge even though it is full of stuff. Some of the stuff is still needed – other stuff is definitely not needed – you need to declutter it – get rid of the rubbish – remove any unnecessary items.

I know you have been thinking a lot about your regrets lately and thoughts have been drifting in and out of your mind. You have also been experiencing so many different feelings too. Thoughts and feelings can serve a purpose. The same could be said of human beings. Through your lifetime you will meet lots of people – some will stay in your life forever – some will be there for a while – others will pass through fleetingly. People come in and out of your life for a reason. It is like friends – you will be friends with people for different reasons – everyone is unique and has something exclusive to bring to a friendship. Some friendships will last forever – others will be time limited. Sometimes it is necessary to declutter people from your life.

It is time to start decluttering. I want you to start making your way around the inside of the shed. Where do you want to start? You will be drawn to places in the shed which contain things you need to declutter. Things that have caused you to have regrets – things that are related to your regrets. Think about your regrets. Think about what you need to declutter – particular thoughts – feelings – behaviours – memories – incidents – situations – people. Start looking around – tell me what you are seeing.

*(Guidance note: at this point the hypnotherapist has to follow the client, because unexpected items can be found. The client will be drawn to areas and objects in the shed. The hypnotherapist may need to encourage the client to open certain things (e.g. boxes; cupboards, drawers) if the object is not immediately visible.*
*Below is a list of prompts and questions which may prove helpful, but the hypnotherapist should use their own questions depending on what is found)*

What have you found?
What are you looking at?
Open that now.
Tell me more about this (*i.e. whatever has been found*).
How are you feeling as you look at/hold this in your hand?
Do you need this in your life now?
Are you ready to declutter it?

*(Guidance note: sometimes the client will say they do not want to declutter an item. When this happens the hypnotherapist needs to explore this further by using the following questions. It may be necessary to return to this item in another session and declutter it at a later stage)*

What is the reason for not wanting to declutter this?
What is the reason for wanting to hold on to it?
What purpose is it serving?
What benefits do you get from this item?

OK so you have found something you want to declutter. Do you want to put it in the skip straight away or are you going to make a pile of things for decluttering inside the shed before you take them outside to the skip?

*(Guidance note: it is best to ask the client first how they want to declutter – what is their own process and preference. They may come up with a unique way of getting things into the skip. Whichever way the client chooses to declutter, the following prompts and questions should be asked as things are put in the skip. If the client has a pile of things to throw in – they should dispose of each item one at a time)*

Pick up *(item for decluttering)* and hold it in your hands.
What are you feeling as you look at it one last time?
Are you ready to put it in the skip?
How will you do this?

*(Guidance note: when the client has finished decluttering it is important to prepare for the future)*

You have done a really good job of getting everything into the skip. You need to go back inside the shed now and just check that there is nothing else that needs decluttering. Then you need to reorganise the inside of the shed. Make sure that everything that is left in the shed is stuff that you really need. You do not want any leftover rubbish. You only need to keep stuff that you know is going to be really useful to you and serve a purpose. Go back in now and have a good look around.

*(Guidance note: if anything else is found which needs decluttering then the process needs to be followed as above)*

Good. Now it is time to reorganise – decide what you want in your life. What do you need in your life? What do you need in your life to make you happy? Think about people – situations – experiences – your personal life – your working life – your hopes – your aspirations – your ambitions. To help you do this, walk around the inside of the shed again and look where you have not looked before. You will find what you need. You will find what will make you happy. Go and look – tell me what you find.

*(Guidance note: the hypnotherapist will work with the client as they find what they need and find a suitable place to store whatever is found. This may take some time if a lot of things are found and it may be necessary to continue in a further session)*

What have you found?
What are you thinking?
How do you feel about finding this?
How will this be useful to you?
Whereabouts will you keep this in the shed?
Do you need to make any more space for this?
Do you need to move anything else around?

Well done. What a good job you have done decluttering in the shed and now it looks so tidy and organised. You know you have everything you need to make you happy and you know exactly where everything is stored. You know you can come back here anytime to do some more decluttering when anything is no longer useful or no longer serves a purpose. From now on you will always remove unnecessary items. You will not hang on to things you do not need. It is now time to leave the shed. Go outside and close the shed door. Look around – you will notice the skip has gone. Now walk slowly back up the garden – as you walk back up – the garden seems wider and more spacious somehow.

# Chapter 41

# Car wash

## Introduction

A visit to the car wash is used to help the client wash away their regrets and the thoughts and feelings associated with those regrets. The regrets are seen in the dirt on the car. There is an emphasis on the fact that dirt, rubbish, scratches and dents can accumulate without even noticing; just like certain thoughts and/or feelings can become the norm in everyday life for a person. The car is cleaned firstly on the outside so it looks clean and polished. Before cleaning the inside, the point is then made that something can look clean and polished on the outside but the inside may look very different.

## The script

You will know that if you have a car you need to service it regularly so that it will continue to run well. It is important that a car mechanic who knows all about cars checks all the parts to see that they are in good working order and to find any faults that might be developing in order to prevent a breakdown. As parts get older they can become faulty and they might need replacing. A car needs various oils and lubricants to keep it running smoothly. It is also important to look after the bodywork of the car and to clean the inside too. You are like a car – you need to be cared for – checked and maintained regularly. Your outside and insides also need to be washed, cleaned and polished. Sometimes it is necessary to wash away dirt and throw away things that have been accumulating – any rubbish that you do not need anymore. You have your own built-in mechanic – your subconscious mind.

Today you are going to go to the car wash. Just imagine a car. Can you see it? Tell me what it is like? *(prompt: make, colour, number of doors etc.)* Now get into the car. You are going to drive to the car wash. Start the engine and off you go. You are driving to a really well-equipped car wash. When you get there you are going to see all the high quality, efficient equipment – high pressure water hoses – hoses for spraying foam car shampoo – buckets – sponges – chamois leathers – cloths – polish – wax machines – hoovers – and anything else you need.

DOI: 10.4324/9781003468325-47

You are pulling up at the car wash now. There are no other customers around. The car wash is for you to use as you wish. You can take as much time as you need to do a thorough wash, clean and polish. Turn off the engine and sit for a while. Think about the regrets that you have – how they have been affecting you – how they have made you feel. It is time now to wash away those regrets – and also the thoughts and feelings that you have been having.

It is time to get the car washed, cleaned and polished. Get out of the car and look at it. Maybe you did not realise how much dirt was on the car. Dirt can accumulate from all different places – as you drive along the road – from all the different journeys you take – when the car is parked up – on a street – in a car park. Dirt can accumulate from all different places – and it can build up without you even noticing. Walk around the outside of the car. Look at the dirt on the car – maybe you see some black marks – dust – leaves – bird droppings – dead insects. You might also notice some scratches on or dents in the paintwork. I wonder if anything has got stuck in the grills on the front of the car or in the tyres. Things can appear and accumulate without you even noticing them.

Just step away from the car now and think about your regrets again. Think about the thoughts and feelings you have been having. Let words float into your mind. Words that you associate with your regrets – words that you associate with the thoughts and the feelings you have. Let words float into your mind. As those words float into your mind see them being written in the dirt on the car. Walk around the car again. See words appearing in the dirt – on the doors – the windows – the bonnet – the boot – the bumpers front and back – and the roof of the car. Look at all the words – keep walking around the outside of the car until the words stop coming into your mind and they stop appearing in the dirt of the car. Tell me when the words stop appearing. Now tell me what words you see written on the car.

*(Guidance note: the hypnotherapist should talk about the words that are in the dirt to understand more about the client's thoughts and feelings)*

Now it is time to clean the car thoroughly – outside and inside. First of all, get the high pressure hose and hose down all the excess dirt off the car. Start to see the dirt and words being removed. Now use one of the hoses to cover the car in foam car shampoo – use as much as you like because you really need to get this car clean and get rid of all the dirt. Do not forget to put some shampoo on the tyres – so much dirt can get trapped in the tyres. They need to be clean and fit for purpose to travel safely. Leave the foam car shampoo for a little while – let it soak into the paintwork and into the tyres. Now it is time to get all the dirt and words removed. Find a sponge and start washing the car. Work on the doors – the windows – the bonnet – the boot – the bumpers front and back – the roof – and do not forget the tyres. Feel the dirt and the words disappearing as you rub hard with the sponge. The dirt is going – the words are becoming fainter and fainter. Keep washing away – the dirt – the words. The words are getting fainter and fainter. Tell me when you have washed them away completely.

Now get the high pressure water hose and rinse the car thoroughly. Tell me when you have finished. Stand back from the car – can you see any dirt or words left on the car?

*(Guidance note: if there is some dirt or words still visible, the hypnotherapist gets the client to repeat the washing process until everything has disappeared)*

Now that the car is perfectly clean you need to dry it off and then you will need to polish the car – make the car shine and sparkle. So get a clean cloth and take off the excess water from the car. Dry it all off. Now you need to polish the car – make the car shine and sparkle. So why not start with the windows first? Find a chamois leather and clean all the windows. You need to be able to see clearly and get a good view out of all the windows – and do not forget the wing mirrors too. You need to have a good view of everything around you – in front – behind – and to the sides. Good job.

Now it is time to polish all the paintwork on the car – the doors – the bonnet – the boot – the bumpers – and the roof. Do not forget the tyres – polish the rims and put some shiny oil on the actual tyres. Keep polishing – make the car shine and sparkle. You notice as you keep polishing that any scratches or dents you noticed before have completely disappeared. The car is looking like new. Keep polishing until you are happy that the car is as shiny and sparkly as you want it to be.

Well the outside of the car is looking great, but I wonder how clean and tidy the inside of the car is. It is so easy to look good on the outside to cover up what is actually going on in the inside. So have a look inside the car. Is there rubbish there – stuff you no longer need? Look on the floor – on the seats – in the cup holders – in the glove compartment – in the side panels of the doors. Make sure you check everywhere – rubbish can fall in between things and get hidden. Put your hand down between and at the side of the seats. Pull out the seat belts. If there is any rubbish – stuff you no longer need – find a black bag and put the rubbish in it. I bet there is all sorts of dirt on the mats and carpets – leaves – soil – stones – grit – empty sweet or chocolate bar wrappers – bits of food – cans – bottles.

So find a hoover and vacuum the inside of the car. It is a powerful hoover – feel the power in your hands as the hoover sucks up the dirt and unwanted things on the mats and carpets. Then hoover the seats thoroughly. OK so now your final task is to polish the inside of the car. There are lots of things that will need a good polish – everything on the dashboard – all the displays – the steering wheel – the instruments – knobs – switches – handles. Polish every surface you can see. Make everything shiny and sparkly.

What a great job you have done at the car wash today. You have washed, cleaned and polished the car thoroughly both outside and inside. You have washed away all the dirt and rubbish you do not need any longer. The car is thoroughly washed, clean and polished. The car is so shiny and sparkly it looks brand new. You and the car are ready to go. Get back in the car – switch on the engine – put the car into gear and off you go. Drive out of the car wash and go in whichever direction you want to take.

# Chapter 42

# Parking the regrets

## Introduction

A car or a van is used in this script to park the regrets, once the client has finished working through them. The concept of the road of regrets is mentioned in the script and the hypnotherapist may want to expand on this whilst using the script, i.e. to review the journey travelled so far in previous sessions.

In the script I have referred to a car being used. However, the client is given the option of driving a van. I have put this into the script because sometimes a client is working on so many regrets and when offered a car to drive away the regrets they say it is not big enough. Therefore, if the client does choose to drive a van the hypnotherapist should use the word van rather than car.

## The script

Today you need to hire a car to transport things you have no further use for in your life. I want you to imagine that you are walking along a street and you are looking for a car hire place. Watch out for a load of cars and vans parked in front of a cabin where the reception area is. Keep walking along until you find it. Tell me when you see it.

Go through the gate and have a walk around the yard. There are a lot of cars and vans – all sizes and different colours. Take your time and have a good look round. I wonder which car or van you would like to drive. Tell me when you have decided. Now go into the reception area and find a person who can help you with all the paperwork and give you the car (*insert van if the client has chosen to drive a van rather than a car*) keys. I shall be quiet for a moment while you sort it out. Let me know when you are ready to go to the car.

Right – go and have a look at the car you have chosen to drive. Tell me what it is like. Have a walk round and become familiar with the outside of the car. Now unlock the driver's door and take a look inside. Become familiar with the inside of the car so you know where everything is and what you have available to drive you in the right direction. Now sit in the driver's seat. Adjust the seat so that you are in

DOI: 10.4324/9781003468325-48

the right position to see clearly out of the windows and so that you feel comfortable. Put the key in the ignition for when you are ready to start the engine.

Look at the dashboard. Put your hands on the steering wheel, which is going to manoeuvre you in the right direction. Now turn the key in the ignition so everything lights up and you can check that everything is in good working order. Test the indicators – because you might need to turn right or left. Find the windscreen wipers and make sure they are working in case it rains – you always need to have a clear view ahead. Also check the windscreen washers in case the windscreen at the front and the rear window get dirty as you travel along. You always need to have a clear view ahead. Now look at the mirrors. Look at the interior mirror and make sure you can see clearly out of the rear window. Then check the wing mirrors – make sure you can see clearly on both sides and behind the car. Finally, just check that all the lights are working.

OK – turn the ignition off again and get out of the car. Walk to the back of the car and open the boot. Look how big it is – very spacious – plenty of room to put things in. Today is the day you are finally going to park your regrets. You have acknowledged them and worked through them. Now it is time to park them up and leave them behind.

For one last time think about your regrets – each individual one you have been working through. As you think about one regret put it in the boot of the car.

*(Guidance note: the hypnotherapist should use the following questions to encourage the client to explain what is happening and how they are feeling as each regret is put in the boot)*

Which regret are you putting in the boot?
What does it look like?
What are you seeing?
What are you thinking?
How do you feel?
Are you ready to put another regret into the boot?

*(Guidance note: the client keeps going until all the regrets have been put into in the boot of the car)*

Are you sure nothing else needs to go into the boot of the car?

OK. Shut the boot of the car and then go and sit in the driver's seat. Make yourself comfortable. Have another look around the inside of the car. You are familiar with all the controls and instruments now which are going to drive you in the right direction. You will not need to use the sat nav or the maps on your phone because you know where you are going – you have an inbuilt instinct of the right way to go – the right direction to take – and the car will take you there. You also have impeccable timing. You know the time is right for a smooth, quick journey without any hold ups. Put your seat belt on. Put the key in the ignition and start the engine. Make your way through the gates of the car hire place and get on to the road. You are nearing the end of the road of regrets. Sit back – relax – you know which way to go to reach your final destination on this road.

Look along the road you are travelling – the road of regrets. You are driving forwards. I wonder what you can see on the road in front of you. I wonder what you can see on either side of the road. You are driving confidently – competently – you know which way to go. Travelling along this road is like travelling through life. Sometimes you have a smooth, uninterrupted journey; at other times you can be held up – when there are a lot of cars, vans and lorries on the road that cause congestion and things move very slowly. Occasionally there can be flooding on the roads after a heavy rainstorm – you can feel like you are drowning in it. Your car can be damaged by potholes in the road. Traffic lights can fail and need to be mended. Any of these events can be a real nuisance and very inconvenient if you are delayed on your journey and sometimes you might miss something important as a consequence. At times you might not be sure of the way to go and can end up going round and round a roundabout several times until you get the right exit. Or maybe you take the wrong turning. None of these things are going to happen today – on this drive. You are driving to your final destination without any delays. Today there is not much traffic on the road – the road is clear – you can travel just as you want to do. Drive at the speed that is comfortable and safe for you. You know exactly in which direction you want to go.

Now you need to start looking for a place where you can park the car and the regrets you no longer want to carry about with you. Keep watching for a multi-story car park – there will be one. Just keep going. Look for a very tall building with a sign saying "Car Parking for Regrets". Tell me when you see it.

Start slowing down and look for the entrance to the car park. You will see a barrier to the entrance. Drive towards it and the barrier will lift automatically. You feel a lightness as the barrier lifts up slowly. Watch the barrier lift up – feel the lightness inside you grow and spread. Drive forward up a ramp. This car park has a lot of floors. It is completely up to you to decide on which floor you want to park the car and the regrets. Take your time there is no rush. Start driving slowing up the ramp and round. Keep driving up – round and round – across a floor. Look for the available spaces. Keep driving up and round – round and round – across the floor. Keep going until you find the right floor to park the car and the regrets. Tell me when you are there. Good – now find the right car parking space. You will find the right car parking space to drive into – it will be big enough and spacious. Tell me when you have found it. Good – now drive into the space and park the car. Make sure the handbrake is on.

Switch off the engine and just sit quietly for a short time. Breathe gently in and out. You know it is time to leave the regrets behind. Today is the day you are finally going to park your regrets. You have acknowledged them and worked through them. Now it is time to park them up for good. Just sit for a while longer – until you feel ready to walk away from the car and the regrets. The regrets have been driving with you for long enough. You need to walk away from them. Just tell me when you are ready.

On the count of *3*, I want you to take the key out of the ignition and get out of the car. *1, 2,* and *3* – get out of the car. Shut the door and lock the car. Now walk away from the car. Breathe gently in and out as you walk away. Walk away from those regrets – breathing gently in and out. Do not look backwards. Keep walking away from the regrets. Find the stairs and walk down the floors until you find the main exit from the car park. Down and down you go – getting further and further away from the car and the regrets you have left behind. Feel that lightness inside you again. As you go down and down the stairs you feel lighter and lighter. Tell me when you have found the exit – left the car park – and you are outside. Take a deep breath in and out. Again – take another deep breath in and out. Start walking and look for a litter bin. When you find one throw the car key into it – and then keep walking.

Now it is time to find a new mode of transport – a vehicle that can drive you towards the future. For now just keep walking towards the future – away from the car park.

Chapter 43

# Visualisations for breaking free and cutting off

## Introduction

Over many years of delivering hypnotherapy sessions I have found that short visualisations can be very effective in getting rid of negative emotions quickly. The overall aim of the visualisations presented below is to help the client break free or cut off from particular emotions which are associated with the regrets they have. A general introduction is included which should be used before using one of the visualisations which are designed to address the following feelings of being:

*   Hemmed in
*   Trapped
*   Tied up
*   Unable to move freely
*   Held back
*   Overwhelmed.

## The script: General introduction for visualisations

Just close your eyes – breathe in and out very slowly – just start to relax. Keep breathing in and out very slowly. Listen to my voice as you continue to breathe in and out very slowly. Having regrets can make you experience all sorts of emotions. You may feel a certain way fleetingly and it will not last long. At other times, the emotional pain might feel like it is never going to go away, but it will go away and I want you to accept this fact. I want you to keep relaxing now – breathing in and out very slowly – going into a deeper trance state. As you are relaxing more now, you are going to think about the emotional pain you have been experiencing and then you will see how it goes away and you will feel different. You will feel a shift deep within you. Keep breathing in and out very slowly.

DOI: 10.4324/9781003468325-49

## 1.   Air raid shelter

You are in an air raid shelter. You are well below ground level but even so you can hear lots of noises – like fireworks – bangs – rockets soaring – screeching – screaming – shouting. You know you are safe here – deep below ground level – but somehow you are still feeling lots of different things which are not comfortable. There are so many people crowded into the shelter. You get the feeling that you know them – you have met them somewhere before. You feel hemmed in – as though you may not get out. You feel trapped and wonder how you would escape if you needed to do so. There are lots of noises above the ground and also below the ground. Noises – voices – all swirling around you – but also feeling like they could be inside you too. Bangs – rockets soaring – screeching – screaming – shouting. Just wait patiently – the noises will stop eventually. There will be no more bangs – rockets soaring – screeching – screaming – shouting. Just bide your time. No more noises above the ground or below the ground. No more bangs – rockets soaring – screeching – screaming – shouting. Just wait patiently – the noises will stop eventually. Listen carefully. The noises are getting quieter – and quieter – and quieter. They will soon stop completely. Everything has to come to an end at some point. You know you can stay with the noises. You can remain calm in this situation. Listen again. The noises are getting quieter – and quieter – and quieter. They have almost gone. Quieter – and quieter – and quieter. Listen again. No noises. People are starting to stand up and move. It is time to leave the shelter. This has been a safe place for you. You may have felt some discomfort but you stayed with those feelings of being hemmed in and trapped. You knew that like the noises those feelings would go away – they would stop. So find your way out of the shelter now. Look forward to breathing in the fresh air above ground level. Find your way out. Up and up you go towards ground level. You are nearly there now. Feel a breeze coming from up above. Smell the air – the freshness. You are nearly there – you can see the sky above – up you go – and you are out.

## 2.   Tied up at the docks

Sometimes you can feel as though you are tied up and you cannot move. You are not being allowed to move freely. Something is holding you back – like a thick rope wrapped around you. Just like when a big ship is moored in the docks. The anchor has been dropped in the water to hold the ship in place; and thick ropes are tied around the bollards which are spread along the docks. The ropes go round and round and round the bollards. Look how tightly the ropes are tied around the bollards. So very, very tight. There is no space between the ropes and the bollards. No room to move. Tied so very, very tight. Restricting the movement of the large ship. The ship cannot go anywhere even though it is so large – much larger than the ropes that are tying it up and so much stronger than the anchor. A man (*use the term woman if the client is female*) comes up to the line of bollards on the dock. He goes to the first one and starts to untie the thick rope. The rope starts to unwind

– unwinding more. The rope is becoming slack – becoming free from the bollard. The ship starts to bob up and down on the water. The man goes to next bollard and starts to untie the thick rope. The rope starts to unwind – unwinding more – becoming slack – becoming free. The ship bobs up and down on the water more quickly. The man then goes to the next bollard. The rope starts to unwind – unwinding more – becoming slack – becoming free. Continue to watch the man as he goes to more bollards and unties all the thick ropes. Unwinding – unwinding – unwinding. The ship is becoming free – free to bob up and down on the water. Free to move just as it likes. Keep watching until all the ropes are untied. Now you see the anchor being brought up out of the water. The ship is now free to set sail and go in any direction it wants. It is no longer restricted by thick ropes or anchored down. The ship is free to travel in any direction it wants.

## 3.   Chopping vegetables

You are in a kitchen standing against a counter. In front of you there is a chopping board and a sharp knife. To the side of the chopping board you see different vegetables – potatoes – carrots – green and red peppers. The vegetables need to be prepared for cooking. Some vegetables need to have the skins removed or bits cut off in order for them to cook nicely. It is important to chop off unnecessary bits – unnecessary bits that make it hard to chew or swallow. You are going to peel the potatoes first. Pick up a potato and hold it firmly in your hand. Feel the texture of the skin. Now start peeling that potato and then peel the other potatoes that are there. Look how easily the skins of the potatoes come off. Keep peeling what is not needed. Now put the carrots on the chopping board. Look at the green leaves on top of the carrots – cut them off. Slice through the top of the carrots. You can do that very swiftly and incredibly quickly – without any hesitation. Now look at the bottom of the carrot – you see the roots dangling – cut them off. You can do that very swiftly and incredibly quickly – without any hesitation. Slice through the bottom of the carrots. You see things can be detached very swiftly and incredibly quickly – without any hesitation. Take the green and red peppers now. Hold them in your hands. Feel how smooth their outsides are. Cut each pepper in half. Look at the insides – see how many seeds there are – all packed together – cramped together. Scrape out the seeds – make the insides of the peppers as smooth as the outsides. Get all the seeds out – scoop them out until the insides are perfectly smooth. Now all the vegetables are prepared.

# Part VII

# Planning for the future

# Chapter 44

# The world is your oyster

## Introduction

This script can be used as an introduction to planning for the future (Stage 5 of the process) or it can be saved for the final session. Most of the work will have been completed, including releasing the regrets and taken any action that was needed. By this stage the hypnotherapist should have an idea about how many sessions might be needed to work on the future. This final part of the process is about focusing on the future, that is, living without the regrets. This script can be used more than once and is a good script to use in a final session to embed optimism and positivity for the future.

## The script

I want to applaud you on how well you have been focusing on and working through your regrets. I think the time has come now for you to look to the future. The time is right to think about how you are going to live your life without those regrets. Think about what you want to do – what you want to achieve. The world is your oyster.

As you are sitting comfortably there, feel proud of yourself. Reflect on what you have achieved over the past weeks/months (*or as appropriate*). Feel really proud of what you have been doing and achieving. You know you can achieve anything you really want to do. The world is your oyster.

I just want you to imagine a coastline somewhere. You are sitting somewhere along a coastline – you can see the sea – it is very close to you. It feels very tranquil here and you feel completely at ease with yourself. Now stand up and walk towards the water's edge – then look down into the water. Keep walking along the water's edge. See if you can find an oyster shell. Keep walking along and tell me when you have found an oyster shell.

Hold the closed oyster shell in one of your hands. Look at the shape of it. Look at the colours on the outside of the shell – maybe some white – grey – or you may see some different colours – purple – pink. Look at the markings on the shell. Use your other hand to feel the shell – you are amazed at how hard and strong the shell is. It protects the oyster inside. An oyster shell can be full of surprises. One always

DOI: 10.4324/9781003468325-51

hopes there will be a pearl inside. A pearl is known as the queen of gemstones – it is a very special gemstone. A pearl can manifest itself in many different ways. You can visualise a pearl in any way you want – whatever is precious to you.

Before you open the oyster shell, I want you to think about what you want for your future. The pearl you want to find in the oyster shell. Your future can be any way you want it to be. Think about what you want to do – what you want to achieve – where you want to go. Remember the world is your oyster.

Now on the count of *3*, I want you to open the oyster shell. It is very firmly closed whilst it is sitting in your hand but in a moment you will prise it open with all your deep inner strength and you will see what you are going to do in the future. Remember you can achieve anything you really want to do. Now on the count of *3 – 1, 2*, and *3* prise open the oyster shell and look inside to your future life. What do you see?

*(Guidance note: the hypnotherapist then works with the client to identify what they want in their future)*

Remember the world is your oyster. You can have the future you want. You will live your future without regrets. You now know what you want for your future. You know you can achieve anything you want to do. You can go anywhere you want to go. Anytime you need to – you can imagine holding the oyster shell in your hand. The oyster shell is hard and strong. You are holding your future in your hand. Look at the oyster shell and know that your own pearl – your own future – is in inside of it. You can open the shell at anytime and look inside – see your future. Remember – the world is your oyster.

Chapter 45

# It's my life

## Introduction

The main script is for clients who have a tendency to put others' needs before their own and then later on in their life they have regrets about doing this. They may even feel guilty about having the regrets; and thinking and feeling the way they do. Even when having these regrets, the person may still carry on in the same way – not thinking about their own needs because they think it would be selfish. Typical examples being:

- Someone who found themselves in the role of a carer, perhaps for a partner or parent, without really having any choice about it.
- A woman who loves her children dearly, but has regrets about having put her career on hold for several years whilst she stayed at home to look after the children.
- A girl who agrees to an arranged marriage to honour her parents' wishes and follow religious/cultural traditions, but has to give up her education and hopes of going to university.

So the aim of this script is to embed the idea that the client and their own needs are important. It is helpful to use the script more than once whilst working on the road of regrets.

Two short additional scripts are included which can be used in conjunction with the main script or in separate sessions. Additional script 1 helps the client to remember times during their life (from childhood through to adulthood) when they were told, pressurised, persuaded or manipulated to do something. Additional script 2 introduces the mantra "It's my life".

## The script

Today I want us to focus on your life and what you want for your future. It is important that you live your life as you wish to do. Through your life you will have had people telling you what to do – what is best you for you – and they might have

DOI: 10.4324/9781003468325-52

said they are telling you for own good. People can tell you what to do with the best of intentions. Parents will have told you what to do when you were a child (and they may still do that now) in order for you to learn and develop. You may have felt at the time it was unjust in what they wanted you to do – like getting homework done rather than being able to go out and play with your friends. However, as you grew up some people may have told you what to do and they may have had their own agenda. This could been done in a very subtle, indirect way – making a suggestion – gentle but repetitive persuasion – so that you did not even realise what was happening. You may have been coerced into doing something.

Sometimes you can feel pressured to do something – do what others want you to do – maybe because of tradition – following a decision made by someone else – which results in taking a certain pathway – or pursuing a certain career in life – or finishing a relationship (*or insert an example the client has talked about from their own life/experience*). Then later you regret it, because you have not followed your heart – your own wishes – your hopes – your aspirations – or your ambitions.

Duty – loyalty – responsibility – can come into play – to make you feel guilty if you do not do something that is expected of you. I wonder if you have felt you have been put under unjust emotional pressure – perhaps what some people might refer to as emotional blackmail.

You have one life – it's your life – and it is important that you live it to the fullest. A caring person will consider other people's needs – and maybe put those needs before their own – perhaps to the detriment of their own needs. Later a person can regret doing that – they feel they have missed out themselves through doing so.

You have the right to live your life as you wish to do. This is a basic human right – as is having choice – being completely free to make your own choices – without any unjust emotional pressure – to help you live your life as you wish to do. It is important to think about yourself – your life – and how you want to live it. This is not being selfish. I wonder how many times someone has told you are being selfish or self-centred when you have decided to do something they did not like – or they did not approve of what you were doing. Remember – you have the right to live your life as you wish to do.

### Additional script 1: To remember the past

Now I want you to focus on your regrets and think about the past. Just let your mind drift back to being a child – a very young child. I wonder how far back you can go. What is your first memory? Then let your mind drift back to being an older child – a teenager – a young person – and into adulthood. Bring forward memories of when you did something because someone told you to do it – or they put pressure on you to do it – or they gently persuaded you – or you felt manipulated somehow. Whatever happened – you felt you did something or perhaps did not do something – that you now regret – because you did not live your life as you wished to do. Perhaps you feel you missed out on an opportunity – an experience – an event – a meeting. Let your mind keep drifting back to being a young child – an older child – a teenager – a young person – an adult. Bring forward your memories. When have you not lived your life as you wished to do?

*(Guidance note: the hypnotherapist will then work to bring forward exact memories/examples of when a person has been made/pressured/coerced to do something)*

### Additional script 2: The mantra – It's my life

Now it is time to focus on your future. Think about what you want for your future. What you want to happen in your life. Remember your life is your life – nobody else's. I want you to say this out loud: It's my life. Say it again: It's my life. Again – say it. One more time. I want you to say this to yourself regularly. You can say it to yourself silently anytime you like – but especially in situations when you feel someone is putting pressure on you to do something you do not want to do. It's my life. So yes you can say it silently: It's my life. As well you can say it out loud – shout it out very loud: It's my life. Do that now – as loud as you can: It's my life. Again – shout it out loud. One more time. How did that make you feel?

Relax now. You know what has happened in the past – you know what you regret. Now focus on the future – what you want to happen in the future.

*(Guidance note: the hypnotherapist will then work to set goals for the future. It is important to see if any of the things which have caused the regrets can be rectified i.e. achieved in the future)*

Is there anything you feel you missed out on that you could be rectified now? (e.g. learning a new skill; training; going for a job/career change)

What do you want to do?
What do you want to experience?

Chapter 46

# Drawing and crossing a line

## Introduction

This script enables the client to leave the regrets behind and move forward into the future, by drawing a line and then crossing it. There is a general introduction to relax the client by focusing on lines and then two additional scripts are presented; the first of which is set on a beach and the second one takes place on a road. The client creates a line and crosses over it leaving the regrets behind and then walks into the future.

## The script: General introduction

There comes a time when enough is enough and it is time to draw a line under something and move on. Do these words sound familiar? Has someone said this to you before? Probably. Drawing a line can be helpful just like crossing a line can be helpful too. So let's do some thinking about lines.

Just relax – let your whole body relax. That's right. Now visualise one straight line – drawn horizontally – look at it from left to right. Then look at it from right to left. I wonder what colour the line is. Look at it again – see how thick or thin the line is.

You know that you have the power to do anything you want. Turn the line around so it becomes vertical. Look at it from the bottom to the top. Then look at it from the top to the bottom. Change the colour of the line. Look at it again – see how thick or thin it is. Now make the line thicker – really make it expand. Now make it go thin again – back to its original size. Now make it go really, really thin until it almost disappears – but it does not disappear. Now return it to its original size. Turn it back to its original colour. Turn it around again so it is horizontal. You see you can do anything you really want to do. You can make changes in your life – you can decide to leave something or someone behind – you can cross a line – you can move forward.

You have been thinking about and doing a lot of work on your regrets. It is time now to leave the regrets behind – draw a line under them – cross over the line and move on with your life.

DOI: 10.4324/9781003468325-53

## Additional script 1: On the beach

Imagine you are standing on a beautiful deserted beach – there is no-one around. The sand is really golden and it stretches far and wide. Look around you – see the sand stretching in front of you. Look behind you – see the sand stretching far into the distance behind your back. Look to the right of you – see how far the sand stretches – look to the left of you – see how far the sand stretches. You may be aware of other things beyond the sand – the sea – the sound of the waves – trees – the sound of birds. For now just concentrate your thoughts on the sand – the beautiful golden sand. Become aware of the sand underneath your feet – between your toes.

Really feel the sand. Now look around you again. Turn towards the direction you want to go – face the direction you know is right for you. You know which direction you need to take, but first you need to do some preparations.

Using your hands and feet, make the sand flat around you – all around you. Use your hands and feet to flatten the area you are standing on – really flatten it – make it really smooth – you know as you flatten it is becoming very sturdy and strong. When that area is really flattened move to your right and again use your hands and feet to make the sand flat around you. Use your hands and feet to flatten the area you are standing on – really flatten it – make it really smooth – you know as you flatten it is becoming very sturdy and strong. You are doing a good job making the sand flat, smooth, sturdy and strong. Now move to the left where the sand is still bumpy and lumpy. You will use your hands and feet again to smooth the sand in the area you are standing on – really flatten it – make it really smooth – you know as you flatten it is becoming very sturdy and strong. Good job.

Look again around you – the immediate area around you – and see how much of the sand has been flattened. If you need to flatten some more of the sand do that now. The flattened area needs to be in front of you – and to your right – and to your left. When you have finished flattening the sand, stand on the sturdy, strong sand. Imagine closing your eyes and taking some really deep breaths. Imagine opening your eyes and on the sand you see a large, thick stick.

Turn around and look behind you – you see the past – you see the regrets you have been working through. Turn around and face forward. Pick up the stick and draw a straight, horizontal line in front in front of you – across the sand – going from right to left and left to right. With the stick draw a very straight line. Make the line as thick or as thin as you like. Make sure the line is straight, sturdy and strong. Tell me when the line is complete – finished just as you want it to be.

Now put down the stick. Keep standing behind the line. Face forward – towards the direction you want to take. Look forward into the distance – see the things you want in your future. Take some deep breaths and focus on the future. Look forward – see what you want to happen. Now it is time to take one last look behind you – you are going to leave the past and your regrets behind you. On the count of *3* you will cross the line and walk into your future. *1, 2,* and *3* – cross the line. Keep walking forward – do not look back – keep walking forward – forward into your future.

## Additional script 2: On the road

Imagine it is early morning. It is just getting light. You are standing on a road – there is no traffic – no people. The road has pavements on either side of it.

Look behind you. You see the road is very uneven. The tarmac is damaged – it is well-worn. You can see lots of potholes – some are very shallow – others are really deep. Now look in front of you and you see that the road is flat. The tarmac on the road is smooth and in excellent condition. Look down at your feet. You see a tin of paint and a big paintbrush.

Take another look behind you. Look at the uneven road. Look at the tarmac – damaged – well worn. Start counting how many potholes you can see. When you have counted the potholes go and take a look down into the potholes. Some will be shallow – others will be very deep. As you look down into the potholes you will see your regrets. Take your time and have a good look at all the regrets you have been working through. The time has come for you to bury the regrets and leave them behind.

On one of the pavements, you notice there are some machines which are for mixing concrete and tarmac. Choose one of the machines and start to create a mixture to fill up the potholes. Set it in motion now. As the machine creates a mixture to fill up the potholes, finish looking down into the potholes. Have one last look at your regrets. The machine stops. The mixture is ready. There is a spade by the machine. Use the spade to fill the potholes. Remember some will be shallow and can be filled up quickly. Others will be really deep and you will need to work hard to fill them. Make sure all the regrets are no longer visible. Tell me when you have finished. Good – now watch as the mixture hardens on top of where the potholes have been. The mixture hardens in the potholes and over the top of them. The mixture becomes hard and strong. The regrets are buried completely.

Now walk away from the filled potholes and the damaged, well-worn tarmac and walk towards the tin of paint and the big paintbrush. Turn to face the part of the road which is flat and where the tarmac is smooth and in excellent condition. It is time to draw a line across the road – you need to leave behind the part of the road which is uneven and where the tarmac is damaged and well-worn. Open the tin of paint and tell me what colour paint is inside. Now pick up the paintbrush and start painting a horizontal line in front of you – across the road – painting from right to left and left to right. Draw the line just as you want it to be. Make the line as thick or as thin as you like. Make sure the line is straight, sturdy and strong. Tell me when the line is complete – finished just as you want it to be.

Now put the tin of paint and the paintbrush to one side. Stand behind the line you have painted on the road. Face forward – ready to walk along the part of the road which is flat and where the tarmac on the road is smooth and in excellent condition. Look forward along the road – see the things you want in your future. Take some deep breaths and focus on the future. Look forward – see what you want to happen. Now it is time to take one last look behind you – you are going to leave the past and your regrets behind you. See that all the potholes have been filled in and the mixture has hardened. On the count of 3 you will cross the line and walk into your future. *1, 2,* and *3* – cross the line. Keep walking forward along the road which is flat – do not look back – keep walking forward – forward into your future.

# Chapter 47

# Galloping and racing into the future

## Introduction

The purpose of this script is to take the client into the future after they have finished working through the regrets by using the image of a racehorse galloping and racing. The script emphasises the importance of preparation to be both physically and mentally strong and embeds motivation and determination to race forward into the future.

I have referred to a male racehorse in the script. If the client is a woman, the hypnotherapist should refer to the racehorse as a female.

## The script

It is time to think about the future and what you want to do in it. You have worked hard on working through your regrets and now you have the future to look forward to – a future without those regrets – the regrets being something you will leave in the past. Now you need to prepare yourself to gallop into the future and enjoy the opportunities that are presented to you.

I want you to imagine a racehorse. A large, strong racehorse. The racehorse is standing very still in a stable. You can see the strong muscles on its body. Look how magnificent the racehorse is. He is standing with his head held high. Look at his four legs – long and strong – able to travel quickly and go the distance. His tail is swishing slightly – ready for the off – he is eager to be off – to race into the future. However, sometimes some preparation is needed before a race starts.

A man walks in carrying horseshoes and a box of tools. He is a blacksmith. He has come to put new shoes on the racehorse. The racehorse is raring to go to start the race – the race into the future – but he needs new shoes – ones which will last him as he goes on his travels and has lots of adventures. So the blacksmith starts to work – one hoof at a time. He takes off the old horseshoe – cleans the hoof – and puts the new horseshoe in position – then hammers in the nails very securely. Just watch as all four horseshoes are replaced – one – two – three – and four. Now the racehorse is physically ready for the race.

DOI: 10.4324/9781003468325-54

The racehorse is looking forward to starting the race – the race into the future. He is prepared physically but he also needs to prepare himself mentally for the race ahead of him. Look at how the racehorse is breathing – slowly and steadily – he is preparing for the start – he is breathing slowly and steadily. He is preparing for the off.

This racehorse is strong and fit. He has been in lots of races and experienced lots of things. He understands how important it is to be prepared – both physically and mentally. He has trained hard to be physically fit – he has built up his stamina. He knows it is also important to have the right attitude – to be motivated – to be determined. He has the desire to win – to be successful. He also knows to do this he has to believe in himself – he tells himself he can win the race. He can go fast – faster than the other racehorses. He can go as fast as he needs to go to win the race.

Watch the racehorse breathing slowly and steadily – preparing himself mentally. He starts to move forward – he walks – he walks quicker – he starts to canter – then he starts to gallop. Watch the horse gallop – galloping – going faster and faster. Look at his head – held high – looking forward – he knows exactly where he is going – going forward. Watch the four legs working together – the muscles are strong and reliable – working together. The racehorse has strength within his body but also strength in his mind. He is going forward with motivation and determination to win. Imagine how the horse feels – feeling that motivation and determination to win.

Imagine you are that racehorse. Galloping into the future. Racing into the future. Feel the determination to go forward and experience new things. You have the physical strength. Feel the strength in your arms – your legs – the trunk of your body – both back and front. You have the physical strength to go forward. Galloping into the future. Racing into the future. You also have strength in your mind. You have the right mental attitude. You are motivated. You are determined. You do not hesitate. You are ready to gallop into your future. You are ready to race into your future.

Think about the things you want to do – the things you want to experience – the things you want to achieve. Imagine them now and gallop along – gallop along towards the things you want to do – the things you want to experience – the things you want to achieve. See them all now. Keep galloping along – feel that motivation deep within you – feel the strength in your body – feel the strength in your mind. Keep galloping along – feel that determination deep within you – feel the strength in your body – feel the strength in your mind. Feel the excitement – you are excited about the things you are going to do – the things you will experience – the things you will achieve – and what you are going to win.

Now it is time to go faster – to really race into your future. So once again think about the things you want to do – the things you want to experience – the things you want to achieve. Imagine them now and race along – go as fast as you can – race along towards the things you want to do – the things you want to experience – the things you want to achieve. See them all now. Keep racing along – go as fast as you can – feel that motivation deep within you – feel the strength in your body – feel the strength in your mind. Keep racing along – go as fast as you can – feel that determination deep within you – feel the strength in your body – feel the strength in your mind. Feel the excitement – you are excited about the things you are going to do – the things you will experience – the things you will achieve – and what you are going to win.

You are nearly there now – at the finish line. You can see it in front of you – your future. Keep racing – go as fast as you can. See the finishing line – see your future. You are nearly there now – going faster and faster – and then you are there – at the finish line. Race over the finish line and you are in your future. You have won the race. Just slow down now – slow down to a canter – slow down some more – and relax. Look at what is in front of you.

# Chapter 48

# Designing a magazine cover

## Introduction

This script should be used when the client is near the end of their treatment plan. The main objective is for the client to consider how they want to be in the future by being both the editor and graphic designer of a brand new magazine. The task is to create a first cover for the magazine that will attract the right readership. This facilitates the client thinking about how they want to be in the future (image) – by considering their values, beliefs and opinions; and who they want to have in their life.

This script can be used in one session and that may be enough for the client to choose the final magazine cover, which will remain as a positive image for the future. However, it may become clear in the early part of the script that the client brings forward a lot of images and this will necessitate the work continuing in another session.

## The script

Designing anything takes thought and time. It is now time to think about you and what you want to design for your future. I want you to imagine that you are the editor of a brand new magazine which is going to be launched in the very near future. You are also a brilliant, creative graphic designer, who can draw any image that comes into your mind and bring it to life.

Imagine that you are in an office that is surrounded by four blank walls. There is a large table in the middle of the room and on it you see lots of drawing materials – pencils – pens – ink – crayons – charcoal – oil paints – paintbrushes. Also there are a lot of sheets of paper on the table – all different sizes – some very big indeed – others quite small – and lots in between. You are the editor of this brand new magazine but you are also going to design the front cover for the magazine because you are a brilliant, creative graphic designer. The magazine is called *(insert first name of client)*. This is a brand new magazine – it has never been published before. The first front cover is very important – it needs to look right – and it also needs to convey the right message concerning what the magazine is about.

DOI: 10.4324/9781003468325-55

Sit down at the table and think about this brand new magazine. What image should it have? Think about its values – beliefs – opinions. What message does it need to give its readers? You want the readership to expand in the future but you also want it to attract the right sort of reader – a reader who understands what the brand new magazine is all about – its values – its beliefs. The right sort of reader will want to read and consider the opinions expressed in the magazine – even if they are different to their own.

So what sort of reader do you want to attract?
Ideally what values and beliefs should they have?
As the editor of the magazine, do you want to express any particular opinions?

So sit now and think about the brand new magazine – the first issue – and the issues which will follow in the future. Let images come into your mind – images you want to create for the first issue of the magazine. Think about you – the editor – the brilliant, creative graphic designer – the brand new magazine. Think about how it will develop in the future – what it will include in the future. I shall be quiet for a short while so you can let the images come into your mind.

*(Guidance note: the hypnotherapist should remain quiet for at least one to two minutes before proceeding)*

It is time to draw those images that have come into your mind. One of those images will become the front cover of the magazine but you do not have to decide which one yet. It would be good to consider all the images before making a decision and then you may want to use some of the other images for the inside of the magazine. You need to draw the images that have come into your head. You are a brilliant, creative graphic designer so you will able to draw any image and develop it until you know it is perfect and exactly how you want it to be. You have plenty of drawing materials – pencils – pens – ink – crayons – charcoal – oil paints – paintbrushes. Also there are a lot of sheets of paper on the table – all different sizes – some very big indeed – others quite small – and lots in between.

*(Guidance note: the hypnotherapist needs to ascertain at this point roughly how many images have come into the client's mind in order to plan whether the work can be completed in this session or whether more sessions will be needed)*

How many images have come into your mind? Bring forward one image. Select a piece of paper from the table and the materials you want to use – then start to draw the image. As you are drawing tell me about the image – tell me about the drawing.

*(Guidance note: the following questions/prompts can be used by the hypnotherapist to elicit information. The hypnotherapist will also use their own questions in response to what the client brings forward)*

What are you drawing?

What is in the drawing?

Are you in the drawing? If yes, how do you look? What are you doing?

Is any other person in the drawing? If yes, who is there? How do they look? What are they doing?

What is happening in the drawing?

What is evolving?

What is the drawing showing?

What is the drawing representing?

How are you feeling as you are drawing?

Tell me when the drawing is complete.

Look at the drawing again. What message is the drawing conveying? What is the drawing saying?

Do you need to do anything else to this drawing – make any amendments/ improvements?

If the drawing is finished, put it up on one of the walls.

Now bring forward another image.

*(Guidance note: the process continues until all the images have been drawn and put up on the walls)*

Now walk around the room. Look at the drawings you have put up on the walls. They are all very good indeed. They convey important messages. Now it is time to choose which one you want to be the first front cover for your magazine. Remember – think about the message you want the brand new magazine to give – and the readership you want to attract. Before making that decision, I want you to think about your future. How you want to be. What you want to happen. Which people – types of person – you want to have in your life – people in your personal life – people in your working life. Think about what you want to do – what you want to experience – what you want to achieve. You know you can do anything you really want to do. You know you can achieve anything you really want to achieve. You can design your life to be just as you want it to be. Think about those things now – think about your future.

*(Guidance note: the client should be given some time to think about this before the hypnotherapist continues with the following questions)*

How do you want to be?

What do you want to happen?

Who do you want in your life?

What do you want to do?

What do you want to experience?

What do you want to achieve?

What will make you happy?

Now look at the drawings on the walls again. Which one will you choose to be the first front cover of your magazine?
Describe the front cover you have chosen to me.
What is the reason for choosing this cover?
What message does the cover convey to the readers?
How do you feel when you look at the first front cover?

Have a look at the other drawings on the walls. Are there any that you would like to include inside this first edition of the brand new magazine?

Now the brand new magazine is ready to go to print. Look at the front cover of the magazine. How impressive it looks. How powerful it is. Flick through the pages inside – look at the articles – stories – information – and messages being given. Look at all the images – illustrations – information – and messages coming together – fixing together – complementing each other. The magazine is now ready to go to print. While it is at the printers it is all coming together – lots of copies being printed through the machines – good clear images – illustrations – articles – stories – information – and messages. The magazine is coming together. The print run is nearly complete. The final copies are being printed. Now the print run is finished. The magazine is ready – ready to be disseminated – and to be read thoroughly and understood.

Chapter 49

# Stained glass windows

## Introduction

This script should be used when the client has worked through their regrets and they are coming to the end of their road of regrets. Stained glass windows one finds in a church usually portray a story from the past. This script takes place in a very old church but is different in that the stained glass windows which are created will tell a story about the client's future.

The hypnotherapist needs to plan for the fact that this work may not be completed in a single session. It may be necessary to keep coming back to create more windows over two or three sessions. It often depends on how much thought the client has given to the detail about how they want their future to be, what they want to do and where they want to go.

## The script

It is time to build a picture of the future – a future without the regrets which have been affecting your thoughts, feelings, how you behave and your life in general. It is time to create a window to the future. A picture which tells the story of your future – how you want it to be. As you are relaxing peacefully there imagine the future. Think about how you want to be – what you want to happen – what you want to do – where you want to go. Just let your mind drift and think about these things – think about your future.

Whilst you are thinking about your future, I want you to imagine that you are in a very old church. You are standing at the entrance and you walk forward towards the aisle. Take a moment and look around you – you see the altar – the stalls where the choir sits – the organ – the lectern from where readings are given – the pulpit from where sermons are given – and the pews where the congregation sits. You do not have to be religious to be here – just enjoy the peace and quiet. Feel at peace with yourself. You have been doing a lot of work on your regrets and now you can feel at peace – at peace with yourself.

You suddenly notice something strange about this very old church. You look at the windows on both sides of the church and you realise that there is no glass in any

DOI: 10.4324/9781003468325-56

of them. Windows need to be made for this church. Stained glass windows can be very colourful and full of brightness. The windows in this church are going to tell the story of your future. Go and sit in a pew for a moment and think again about your future – how you want to be – what you want to happen – what you want to do – where you want to go. I am going to be quiet for a short while so you can think about these things – how you want to be – what you want to happen – what you want to do – where you want to go.

*(Guidance note: the hypnotherapist should remain quiet for one to two minutes)*

Now go and have a look at the back of the church where you will find all the things you need to make some stained glass windows – glass – glass cutters – tape measure – ruler – paint – paint brushes – putty – glue – sealant – and anything else you might need. Each stained glass window that you make is going to tell the story of your future. Feel the excitement growing inside of you. You are the creator – the artist – who has lots of skills – you can cut out the future you want for yourself.

Now think about the first window you want to make. What is it going to show? What story does it need to tell?

*(Guidance note: the hypnotherapist should encourage the client to describe what aspect of the future is to be shown. The following questions can be used as prompts if required)*

What will be in the window?
Will any person/people be in the window?
What do you want to see in the window?
What do you want to show in the window?
What story is going to be told in the window?

Now get the materials ready and set to work. Remember you are the creator – the artist – who has lots of skills – you can cut out the future you want for yourself. Choose one of the empty windows – a space where you want to put in a stained glass window. Look at the shape of the window – measure it accurately so the stained glass window will fit perfectly. Then get the glass you need and cut it as required to fit the window. It will be a perfect fit because you have measured the space accurately. Now think about what you want to draw and paint onto the glass. Think about story you want to tell about the future.

*(Guidance note: the hypnotherapist should ask the client to describe what they are doing/making as the window is created. The following questions can be used as prompts if required)*

I am interested to know what you are creating.
Tell me what you are doing.
What are you doing with the glass?
How are you cutting the glass?
What shape will the glass be?
What are you drawing?
What are you painting?
Describe the picture to me.
What is being shown in the window?
How are you feeling as you are creating this window?
Let me know when the window is finished.

Now place your stained glass window in the empty space you have chosen and measured accurately. Place the glass securely in the space – it will fit perfectly, because you know exactly how it should be. Then you need to fix it permanently – remember you have putty – glue – and sealant to do this. Make the stained glass window really safe and secure. Now stand back – away from the stained glass window. Look at it – what are you seeing? What are you feeling? Now tell me the story which is told in the window.

*(Guidance note: the client will tell the story)*

Would you like to make another stained glass window?

*(Guidance note: the hypnotherapist should then repeat the process to create another stained glass window. Sometimes all the windows can be completed in one session. However, it may be necessary to do this work over more sessions)*

# Part VIII

# Additional scripts

Chapter 50

# Freya the fox and the eggs

## Introduction

I wrote this script specifically for children who have some regrets and feel guilty about having done something that they did not realise was wrong. I also wanted to address the issue of saying sorry or showing you are sorry. This script can be used with any child from the age of 5 upwards. The hypnotherapist may wish to adapt the language in the script to make it age appropriate for the child/young person.

## The script

Sometimes we can do things that we think are alright – we do not realise that what we are doing is wrong – but in fact it is not a good thing to do or not the right thing to do. A person can regret what they did when they do realise this and feel very sorry for having done what they have done. It can be important to try to put things right – a starting point is to say sorry and mean it. I know you regret/feel sorry about (*insert what the child regrets*), so that is why I would like to tell you about a young fox cub called Freya.

I am not sure how much you know about foxes. They are usually born in March or April and they live with their parents in what is called a den. The parents look after the fox cubs in the den until they are about six weeks old. Then they are allowed to go out of the den and explore the area with their parents, who teach them lots of different things. The parents teach the cubs how to survive – how and where to look for food. Then when the cubs are about two months old they are allowed to go out by themselves.

Freya was a red fox, who lived with her mum and dad and two brothers. She was very excited about going out to find food on her own. Freya lived in a big city and sometimes it can be really hard for foxes to find enough food to survive. There are so many foxes roaming the streets in the city and they all have their own routes. Foxes are creatures of habit – they like to travel the same way at the same time each day – well actually it is usually at night or very early in the morning. Freya had gone out with her parents and brothers all together; and she had also gone out with her mum – just Freya and her mum – the girls together. She learnt which route

DOI: 10.4324/9781003468325-58

her mum took every night. Freya had got to know her mum's route – the roads – the gardens – the back yards – the fences to climb – the trees to hide behind – the garage roofs to cross over. Her mum had taught her how to be safe. Freya was confident she knew where to go and what to do.

So the first night Freya went out by herself she explored a few streets she knew and then because she was a very curious fox she decided to find some new streets. She was just going up one street when she heard banging and clattering. There were sounds she was not familiar with at all. She crept up slowly to a large van that was parked in the middle of the street. The van had crates of milk bottles and boxes of other things on the back. A man got out of the van and grabbed a crate of milk bottles. Freya watched him carefully as he went to different houses and left milk bottles on the doorsteps. She thought that was a strange thing to do. The man then came back to the van, placed the empty crate on the back and picked up a big box. He then went to more houses where he took out funny looking small boxes from the big box and left them on the doorsteps. Again Freya thought this was a strange thing to do. The man then got back in the van and drove off.

As I have said before, Freya was a very curious fox so she decided to go and look at what the man had left on the doorsteps. She sniffed at the objects – the milk bottles – the funny looking boxes – and some other things. Freya liked the look of the funny looking boxes which were in fact egg boxes. She poked her nose around one box and ripped it open with her strong teeth. She had never seen an egg before. So she sniffed each egg and then bit into one of them. She licked the liquid inside. She absolutely loved the taste. She sucked out the liquid and ate everything that was inside of that egg. She kept licking the inside of the shell to make sure she had not left any of the delicious tasting stuff. She went on to bite open some more eggs – sucked out the insides of the eggs and ate them – and then licked the insides again. Freya loved eggs from that night – and from then on she went out and ate eggs every night. Freya developed her own route – going to the streets where the man delivered the eggs.

The people on the streets in the area started complaining to the milk company who not only delivered milk and eggs but also lots of other things too – cream – fruit juices – yoghurts – butter. The people on the streets complained that they were either not receiving the eggs they had ordered or the eggs were cracked. Also they were finding empty egg boxes and egg shells on their doorsteps, in their gardens and on the street. It was all looking very untidy. The milk company thought it was very odd that all the complaints they were receiving were about eggs – not about the milk, fruit juices, yoghurt, butter or other products. The people on the streets did not understand what was happening and the milk company did not understand either.

So this went on for a few weeks. Then one night a man called Jack went out to call his two cats in for the night. It was actually very late at night. Jack was calling out to the cats and as he walked around the garden he suddenly saw something move. He thought it was the cats – but it was not. He saw a big bushy tail – a tail much bigger than a cat's tail. There was movement again and suddenly he saw the face of a fox, with liquid dripping from its mouth. It was Freya – she had been eating eggs again. The mystery was solved. Jack in a firm voice told the fox to "Go away and don't steal our eggs anymore". Freya was a bit confused – "What is an egg?" she thought.

Freya went home and asked her mum what an egg was and explained what had happened. Freya's mum explained what an egg was and how the boxes of eggs left on doorsteps belonged to the people living in the houses. What Freya had been doing was stealing the eggs. Freya felt terrible when she heard this and started to regret finding the new streets and forming a new route. Her mum explained very clearly that it was not her fault because Freya was a young fox cub and still learning right from wrong. She did not know what an egg was and she did not know the eggs in the funny looking boxes belonged to someone else. Freya said she was really sorry about what she had done. Freya's mum said Freya needed to do something to show she was sorry and she had an idea about how Freya could do that.

That night, Freya and her mum went out on Freya's route. Freya's mum said it would be good to tidy up the litter on the doorsteps – in the gardens – and on the streets. There was a lot of litter about on the doorsteps – in the gardens – and on the streets – including empty egg boxes and lots of egg shells. Freya and her mum spent the whole night tidying up all the litter – not just the empty egg boxes and the egg shells. By the time they had finished all the streets looked so tidy and clean. When the people on the streets woke up the next morning and went outside they could not believe how tidy everywhere was – and that is how it stayed.

Freya had felt sad for a while after she had found out she had been stealing and she regretted what she had done. Her mum explained it was not her fault and said some very wise words: "We all make mistakes. We all have to learn and we can learn from our mistakes. It is also important to say sorry if you can and if you cannot put sorry into words then doing something – taking action – to show you are sorry is just as good. Actions can sometime speak louder than words". And Freya's mum was right, wasn't she? Freya felt so much better when she had tidied up the streets to show she was sorry.

# Chapter 51

# Sophia the seamstress

## Introduction

This metaphorical script is for clients who are experiencing guilt because they feel they have failed to keep someone safe and/or they could not persuade someone to leave a bad situation (in this case a domestic abuse situation). Sophia uses her imagination as a distraction in childhood when living in poverty and witnessing her mum being abused by her father. The coping strategies she develops in adulthood whilst working as a seamstress can be used for (and taught to) the client.

## The script

Sophia is a very successful seamstress. She has made beautiful clothes for lots of people over the years. Sophia did not have an easy childhood. She heard and saw many things no child should ever witness. Her life was very chaotic way back then. Her dad drank a lot and often failed to bring money home, so Sophia and her mum were regularly left without food and the house was very cold. Children at school made fun of Sophia's clothes, which were very old and worn. Sophia often wanted to run away from home, but she felt she could not leave her mum. She pleaded with her mum to leave her dad, but her mum refused to do so. She used to say: "I've made my bed I have to lie in it". Sophia was determined that she would never let anyone control her once she left home. She used to daydream about leaving home and having a job, but then she felt guilty about having these thoughts. As soon as she could leave school, Sophia did. She wanted to have a trade and she chose to be a seamstress so that she could make clothes for herself – as well as others – and so no-one would ever make fun of her again. She got an apprenticeship and learnt how to design and make clothes. She continued to live at home and only left when her mum died.

I am telling you about Sophia, because she had many regrets – regrets about not having what she called "a proper childhood". She also felt guilty that she had not protected her mum from the violent beatings she received from her dad, but in fact there was nothing she could have done about that. She regretted not leaving home before she did. When Sophia lived at home she spent a lot of time imagining how

DOI: 10.4324/9781003468325-59

life could be different – what she could do – where she could go. I want to tell you more about this.

Sophia would sit with her eyes closed and imagine an item of clothing – maybe a beautiful dress – blouse – skirt. She would see the colours – and imagine feeling the fabric. She would sit like this for a while. When she opened her eyes she would take some tissue paper, a pair of scissors and cut out the shape of the item of clothing. She would then source the fabric and when she had it in her possession she would pin the tissue paper to the fabric and cut out the shape of the item. She took her time doing this as she did not want to make any mistakes. She did not want to waste any fabric.

Sophia would then prepare the sewing machine with the right colour thread and then she would put the garment together. Sophia felt calm when she was making things. Focusing on what she was doing engrossed her – took her away from what was happening in her house. She found it calming when she was flattening out the fabric – making it smooth. She felt creative when she pinned the tissue paper and fabric together – she could see a garment taking shape. She made things firm – permanent – when she used the sewing machine. She liked the speed and the firmness of the machine. She also liked to sew by hand. Pulling the needle and thread in and out of the fabric made her feel calm – in and out – in and out. Sometimes when her minded drifted into a trance whilst she was sewing, she became so relaxed she forgot what she was doing and pricked her finger. That sometimes happens in life, everything is going well and then something happens which you do not expect and you experience pain.

Other sewing methods helped Sophia too. She found she could stop intrusive thoughts – or feeling a certain way – when she bit off or cut through some thread with scissors. She imagined pushing thoughts and feelings she did not want to have into a pocket or up a sleeve. She loved ironing a finished garment to press down her thoughts and feelings. She could put an end to something by pulling a zip upwards. All these things helped Sophia cope with the thoughts and feelings she experienced. These were her coping strategies.

Sophia was very creative and also very methodical – she liked to have a system in place to make her feel safe and secure. This was because her life at home through childhood and into adulthood had been so chaotic. She never knew if she was going to being fed – what mood her dad would be in – whether her mum would be hurt. When she left home she was determined to feel safe – she wanted to have a secure income – she wanted to be warm – she wanted to have regular meals. She wanted to be happy.

For a long time after her mum died Sophia had regrets. She wished she could have persuaded her mum to leave her dad. She wondered if she had been able to do that whether her mum would have lived longer and had a happier life. It was not Sophia's fault that her mum believed she had to stay in that situation. Sophia did have regrets but once she worked her way through them she became a very successful seamstress. People loved the garments she made for them; and so they kept coming back for more. Sophia had achieved what she wanted – she felt safe – she had an income – she was warm – she had regular meals – and she was happy.

So let's think about you now and how you feel. Maybe you could use some of Sophia's sewing methods to help you cope. Is there anything you want to:

Bite or cut off
Push into a pocket or up a sleeve
Iron to press things down
Put an end to by pulling a zip upwards?

Chapter 52

# Not having a childhood

## Introduction

Childhood should be a time in life when you are carefree, happy and have a sense of freedom to explore, experiment and live life to the full. Unfortunately, this is not what some children experience. Many children in the UK are what we now refer to as a "young carer", i.e. they are responsible for caring for someone else in the household. That person could be a family member, a friend or someone else who lives in the house; and that person could have an illness, a disability, a mental health problem or an addiction to drugs or alcohol. The young carer provides both practical and emotional support and assistance. Statistics regarding how many young carers there are can differ tremendously depending on the ages researched (e.g. is a young carer under 25 or under 18 years of age?) and who is actually undertaking the research. Whatever research we are considering, the statistics are depressingly high. The Children's Society states the following as facts regarding young carers in England[1]:

- There may be more than 800,000 young carers
- Carers could be as young as 5 years old
- 27% of young carers aged 11 to 15 years miss school
- 1 in 3 young carers have a mental health issue.

A person who been a young carer can feel in adulthood that they never had a childhood – they were robbed of it. The emotions experienced both in childhood and adulthood can become very complicated and entwined. Consequently, such an adult can seek help from a hypnotherapist. Very often they have regrets emanating from the fact they feel they never had the experiences a child should have in childhood. The metaphor which follows tells the story of Julie, who had very conflicting emotions regarding her mum: love; care; loyalty; duty; responsibility; hate; anger and resentment.

DOI: 10.4324/9781003468325-60

## The script

I want to tell you about a woman called Julie, because I think you may be able to understand and relate to her situation. I also think you can learn from what happened to her.

When she was a child, Julie lived with her mum and two younger brothers. Her Dad had died when she very young and she does not remember anything about him. Her mum, Christine, felt lost when Julie's dad died and she started drinking more than she usually did. Christine had lots of family living nearby. None of them worked and they used to spend all day, every day, at each others' houses. Christine started getting into a lot of debt, because she was drinking so much. She did not pay the bills and very often there was no food in the house.

Julie really took over her mum's role. In the morning, Christine would be fast asleep and Julie would wake up her brothers, get them ready for school and then the three of them would walk to school together. They were often starving when they arrived at school because there had been nothing to eat in the house for breakfast. This became a regular occurrence and the three children would be so hungry until lunchtime when they got a free school meal. There were no breakfast clubs way back then. Julie felt it was her responsibility to look after her two little brothers, but also her mum. So Julie started stealing food from the local corner shop. She never got caught.

Birthdays and Christmases were miserable times. Julie used to say: "All I want is a doll. A beautiful girl doll". She never got one. Christine did not have any money for presents and her extended family also had financial problems of their own, so there were no presents for anyone.

Julie started to become angry. She grew into being a very angry teenager. She loved her two brothers without a doubt, but she had mixed feelings about her mum. Julie said: "One half of me loves my mum; the other half hates her". Julie could never let go of the fact: "I never had a childhood. All I wanted was a girl doll".

As you might expect, Julie ended up in a lot of bother in her teens. She carried on stealing; she got into fights and she was arrested several times. So you may be wondering what happened to Julie and where she is now. She is now a woman in her 50s, who has a huge collection of dolls. She had kept being an angry teenager until Christine died of liver failure when Julie was 19 years old. Something suddenly changed for Julie then. She had left school when she 16 years old and had lots of different jobs, but did not stick at any of them for very long. She also found it difficult to maintain relationships. The only people she really loved were her brothers and she felt she had a responsibility to look after them anyway she could.

Julie said she felt a sense of release when her mum died and that is when she decided that she had to do something with her life. She decided to go to college to study. It was one of the tutors who referred Julie to a therapist so she could work through the anger and resentment she felt towards her mum. She resented the fact she had never had a childhood. She regretted that she had never been able to do what she considered to be "normal things as a child" – and that she had never had a "girl doll". In the therapy sessions she also talked about regretting stealing and being violent.

Therapy helped Julie. She talked through her feelings and about her regrets. Part of the work which was done included Julie making a list of all the things she felt she had missed out on because she believed she had never had a childhood. She then did those things as an adult. There were all sorts of things written on the list – some things many people might take for granted – like (and these are Julie's words):

- Going to see a film at the cinema
- Eating a Happy Meal in McDonald's
- Going to see the seaside/swimming in the sea/making sandcastles
- Having a Christmas stocking at the end of my bed/Christmas presents
- Having a birthday party/birthday presents
- Being read to
- Always having food in the house
- Being able to buy an ice-cream from the ice-cream van that comes on the street
- Having a picnic
- Being warm/the gas and electric never being cut off
- Having clean clothes that are ironed.

Julie felt bad that she had regularly stolen from the local shop when she was really young. The shop owner still had the shop so Julie went to talk to him about what she had done. He said he had known what was she was doing but understood the situation she had been in so ignored her stealing food from the shop.

After college Julie went to work as an administrative assistant in a local nursery. She loves children but has never had any of her own. Once she was in a permanent job and had a steady income, she started to buy dolls – and she has continued to collect dolls ever since. So now she has a wonderful, huge collection of girl dolls.

So shall we think about you now?

## Note

1  https://www.childrenssociety.org.uk/what-we-do/our-work/supporting-young-carers/facts-about-young-carers

# Chapter 53

# On the motorway

## Introduction

This script works nicely with the concept of travelling along the road of regrets. It can be used over several sessions to go on different journeys; and it can be used at different stages of the process. Hence its inclusion in Part VIII. It will be necessary to highlight what action needs to be taken in regard to the regrets and each action can be dealt with on a separate journey. The *Ending* section can be used at the end of each journey taken or just as a short script for the final drive away from the regrets in order to leave them behind forever. Alternatively, the hypnotherapist might choose to use the script for the sole purpose of driving into the future.

## The script

Some people like driving on motorways – others do not. A motorway is usually a more direct route to where you want to go. Also it is often much quicker, unless there are roadworks or an accident has occurred which holds you up. Lots of things can happen in life which hold you up and being slowed down can be very inconvenient.

Today you are going to drive on a motorway. Imagine yourself in a car – driving competently and confidently. You are in the lane nearest the hard shoulder. It is not very busy. You are cruising along steadily at 70 mph. Have a look around you – be aware of the cars around you. Look at the cars in front of you – in all of the three lanes. Then look to see if there are any cars to the side of you. Use your mirrors – rear view mirror and the wing mirrors – to see the cars that are behind you in all three lanes. You always need to be aware of what is going on around you and what is happening near you – in front of you – behind you – to the right of you – and to the left of you. People can do things unexpectedly which can have an impact on you. Things can happen which are not your fault at all. Watch out for any cars that are going too fast – coming up to overtake you – you do not want any surprises.

Today you are going to find a new route that will eventually take you into your future leaving your regrets behind forever. In order to do that you need to steer away from the regrets that have been holding you back. It is very easy to drive the same route every day and not be very observant. You may not really take any

DOI: 10.4324/9781003468325-61

notice of what is happening because you take things for granted as you see the same things every day. Things around you feel familiar. Everything is in its place. Or maybe you think there is no other route to take. Taking the same route every day is comfortable – it is easy – you know what you are doing.

This motorway is going to take you in a new direction. You are going to leave your regrets behind and drive into the future. As you continue to drive along the motorway competently and confidently, I want you to start thinking about whether there is anything you need to do before you leave the regrets behind for good. Think about whether you need to drive somewhere to:

Have a conversation with someone
Explain something to someone
Say sorry
Make amends
Ask someone a question(s)
Find someone
Find out what happened
Find out the truth.

What do you need to do?
Where would you like to drive to?

*(Guidance note: usually the client will want to do something and drive somewhere to take action. If this is the case the hypnotherapist will continue with the script and may choose to use another script to achieve an objective before coming back to the end of this script)*

So this is the start of an important journey. How many junctions do you need to travel to get there? Keep driving on the motorway and tell me when you have reached the junction where you need to exit. Good – take the exit now and drive to the destination where you need to (*insert whatever the client has chosen to do*).

*(Guidance note: use another script to work on the action to be undertaken/ an objective e.g. plan a meeting)*

## 1.  Ending

You are back on the motorway now. Well done; you have achieved a lot on this journey. Do you think there are any more journeys you need to take to sort things out before leaving your regrets behind forever?

*(Guidance note: if the answer is yes then another journey can be taken in the same session or the script can be used again in the next session. Once a client has done everything they need to do, which may involve several journeys, the final journey can be taken and completed)*

## 2.  *The final journey*

Keep driving along the motorway for now. Concentrate on driving away from your regrets because you have dealt with them. You have done everything you need to do. It is time to drive forward to your final destination – a place where you have no regrets. Keep driving. You are driving competently and confidently. You feel calm and relaxed. Looking forward to reaching your final destination – a place where you have no regrets. You are in the lane nearest the hard shoulder. It is not very busy. You are cruising along steadily at 70 mph. Have a look around you – be aware of the cars around you. Look at the cars in front of you – in all of the three lanes. Then look to see if there are any cars to the side of you. Use your mirrors – rear view mirror and the wing mirrors – to see the cars that are behind you in all three lanes. Keep driving. You are driving competently and confidently. You feel calm and relaxed. You are looking forward to reaching your final destination – a place where you have no regrets.

So it is time to get there. You need to change lanes. Indicate and drive into the middle lane and while still indicating drive into the fast lane. Now really go for it – drive as fast as you can to your final destination. Look in the rear view mirror – see all your regrets being left behind. You are speeding away – the regrets become smaller and smaller as they go further and further into the distance behind. The regrets are becoming smaller and smaller. Keep driving until you cannot see them at all. Tell me when you cannot see them any longer.

They have gone – you have left your regrets behind forever. Slow down a bit now. You are feeling calm and relaxed. You need to change lanes again. Indicate and drive into the middle lane and still indicating drive into the slow lane. Just take your time enjoying the rest of the journey. Think about the future. Look forward to the future. Drive towards your future. Drive along – see the future in front of you. Tell me what you see.

Chapter 54

# Rowing

## Introduction

Rowing is another way of travelling along the road of regrets (or in this case a lake). The main purpose of this script is to build determination and strength by rowing a boat on a lake. If required, the script can be used soon after introducing the concept of the road of regrets. It can be beneficial to use the script in several sessions at different stages of the process. Alternatively, it can be used once in a later session to get the client to row to their final destination. A shorter alternative version of the script is also presented which can be used early on in the therapeutic process (Stage 2) to regress a client to a time or event that has been significant in causing the regrets, which have already been identified and acknowledged in Stage 1 of the process.

## The script

Today you are going to go rowing – rowing in a boat. Rowing a boat on a lake can be such a pleasant way to spend some time relaxing. It can be a really good way of exercising your body and exercising your mind – rowing can also have another purpose. It can build up your determination and strength. The people who row in teams have to train hard individually and as a group. They need to be physically fit and mentally fit. They have to work together and synchronise their movements as they pull the oars in and out of the water. Their arms and legs need to be very strong. The way a team works is very much like how you and your subconscious mind work together. If you are determined to do something – you will do it – you can achieve it – anything is possible. You have strength embedded deep within you already but you can build on that strength so it becomes stronger and stronger.

So imagine that you are walking down a path towards a lake. It is a bright sunny day and you feel a gentle breeze as it brushes across your face. Notice the trees around you as you walk down the path towards the lake. See branches and leaves on the trees being blown gently by the breeze. You may hear some birds singing. You may see some herons or other birds hunting for fish or other food they enjoy. You may hear the water moving on the lake. As you get nearer to the lake you see

DOI: 10.4324/9781003468325-62

a boat sitting on the water. It is swaying gently side to side. Watch the boat swaying side to side – it is so relaxing – swaying side to side. You are relaxing more and more as you watch the boat swaying side to side. You are getting near to the water's edge now. You need to untie the boat and get into it. You will find two oars in the boat, which you can use to steer the boat in the right direction.

You are now sitting in the boat. Make yourself comfortable. Pick up the oars – take one in each hand and place the blades in the water. Grip the oars tightly in each hand. Think about which direction you want to take. Then think about how you will row this boat. Imagine holding and pushing the oars in and out of the water. Imagine your legs and knees pushing backwards and forwards. Feel the strength in your hands – wrists – lower arms – elbows – and upper arms. Feel the strength in your feet – ankles – calves – knees – and thighs. Feel the strength in the trunk of your body – in your stomach – in your back – in your shoulders – and neck. Feel the strength in your mind. Feel the determination to row in the right direction. You are ready to row.

Push the boat away from the side and start rowing the boat on the lake. Nice and slowly to begin with – there is no need to rush. Just enjoy moving on the lake. Feel the gentle swaying of the boat as you row – you get into a rhythm. Using your arms – lifting the oars up and down through the water – using your legs – pushing backwards and forwards. That is right – getting into a rhythm. Using your arms – lifting the oars up and down through the water – using your legs – pushing backwards and forwards. Enjoy the movement – the swaying.

You know which direction you want to take. You can go in whichever direction you know is right for you. You can row slowly or quickly. It is up to you how quickly you want to reach your destination. For now though keep rowing gently – build up your strength slowly.

Members of a rowing team have to build up their strength for the races they will participate in. It takes time for strength to develop in the different parts of the body. Feel the strength building in your hands – wrists – lower arms – elbows – and upper arms. Feel the strength building in your feet – ankles – calves – knees – and thighs. Feel the strength building in the trunk of your body – in your stomach – in your back – in your shoulders – and neck. Feel all the muscles in your body getting stronger and stronger. The more rowing you do the stronger your body will become.

Rowing does not just strengthen your body – rowing can strengthen your mind. The more rowing you do – the more determined you will become. I know you are determined to get to your destination. You have the right attitude – you want to succeed – you know you can succeed – you know you will succeed – because you are determined to do so. Feel that determination growing. Feel the determination in your mind. You have so much determination and strength in both your mind and body. Keep rowing – it is such good exercise for your mind and body.

So now go a little faster. Pull harder on the oars – in and out of the water. The blades dip in and out of the water more quickly now. Feel the strength building in your hands – wrists – lower arms – elbows – and upper arms. Feel the strength building in your feet – ankles – calves – knees – and thighs. Feel the strength building even more in the trunk of your body – in your stomach – in your back – in your shoulders – and neck. Feel all the muscles in your body getting stronger and stronger. The more rowing you do the stronger your body will become.

Now go even faster – going faster and faster on the water. Skimming over the lake. Passing swiftly over the water – going faster and faster. Even faster and faster. Your body is working well – it is powerful – it is growing in strength – and it will continue to do so. Your mind is working well – it is powerful – it is growing in strength – and it will continue to do so. Feel that determination deep within you – it is growing – and it will continue to do so. So keep rowing until you get to where you want to be. You are getting near your final destination. Nearer and nearer now – you are almost there. You can see your final destination – keeping rowing – almost there – and then you are there. How does it feel to have reached your final destination?

## Additional script: Rowing to regress

Today you are going to go rowing – rowing in a boat. Rowing a boat on a lake can be such a pleasant way to spend some time relaxing. It can also be a really good way of exercising your body and exercising your mind – also rowing can also have another purpose. It can take you back in time.

So imagine that you are walking down a path towards a lake. It is a bright sunny day and you feel a gentle wind as it brushes across your face. Notice the trees around you as you walk down the path towards the lake. See branches and leaves on the trees being blown gently by the breeze. You may hear some birds singing. You may see some herons or other birds hunting for fish or other food they enjoy. You may hear the water moving on the lake. As you get nearer to the lake you see a boat sitting on the water. It is swaying gently side to side. Watch the boat swaying side to side – it is so relaxing – swaying side to side. You are relaxing more and more as you watch the boat swaying side to side. You are getting near to the water's edge now. You need to untie the boat and jump into it. You will find two oars in the boat, which you need to steer the boat back in time.

You are now sitting in the boat. Make yourself comfortable. Pick up the oars – take one in each hand and place the blades in the water. Grip the oars tightly in each hand. Think about which direction you want to take – you are going to row back in time. Think about how you will row this boat. Think about holding and pushing the oars in and out of the water. Imagine your legs and knees pushing backwards and forwards. Feel the strength in your hands – wrists – lower arms – elbows – and upper arms. Feel the strength in your feet – ankles – calves – knees – and thighs. Feel the strength in the trunk of your body – in your stomach – in your back – in your shoulders – and neck. Feel the strength in your mind. You have the ability to row back in time.

So now you are ready – ready to row back in time. Push the boat away from the side and start rowing the boat on the lake. Nice and slowly to begin with – there is no need to rush. Just enjoy moving on the lake. Feel the gentle swaying of the boat as you row – you get into a rhythm. Using your arms – lifting the oars up and down through the water – using your legs – pushing backwards and forwards. That is right – getting into a rhythm. Using your arms – lifting the oars up and down through the water – using your legs – pushing backwards and forwards. Enjoy the movement – it is so relaxing – swaying side to side. Relaxing more and more as you row back in time

Keep rowing; nice and steady. As you push the oars in and out of the water the boat is moving backwards. Going backwards – backwards through time. Keep rowing – nice and steady. Going backwards – backwards through time. Although you are looking forward you know you are rowing backwards through time. You are rowing through the years and the decades you have lived – backwards and backwards – backwards through time. You will keep rowing – moving backwards – back as far as you need to go to a time that has caused you to have regrets. Keep rowing – moving backwards – back to the time you need to go to – to a time that has caused you to have regrets. Getting nearer now – keep rowing – you sense you are nearly there – back to the time you need to go to – to a time that has caused you to have regrets. Tell me when you are there. Get out of the boat – tie up the boat. Walk now – into the time – the time that caused you to have regrets.

*(Guidance note: the hypnotherapist will then help the client to relive and work through the significant time/events which have caused the regrets)*

Chapter 55

# The computer screen

## Introduction

This script works well for any child or adult who likes being on a computer. If the hypnotherapist knows the client uses an Ipad a lot, then the word Ipad can be substituted for computer. The idea is for the client to write words or draw things on the screen to express how they feel about their regrets. They also take a look at themselves via the webcam. Those pages are eventually deleted. Pages are also created about the future by writing or drawing. Those pages are saved. The client then takes another look at themselves via the webcam to see the changes in themselves.

## The script

Make yourself comfortable and imagine that you are looking at a computer screen. You have logged into a very special programme. Look at the screen. It looks as though there is a blank sheet of white paper on the screen. At the bottom of the screen you see there is a toolbar – one you have not seen before. So you need to learn about all the wonderful things it can do. It is time to undertake some experimentation.

So focus your attention on the toolbar at the bottom of the screen. At each end of the toolbar there is an arrow. The one on the left hand side will let you go backwards. The one on the right hand side will let you go forwards. Next to the arrow on the left hand side there is an icon that looks like a pencil. By clicking on the pencil icon with the mouse, you can use the pencil to write or draw. If you keep clicking on the pencil you will see that it can change to write and draw in many different colours. Keep clicking and then choose a colour you would like to write in. Now think about the regrets you have and how they have been making you feel. Click on the pencil and write some words down that come into your head as you remember how you have been feeling about your regrets. Tell me what words you are writing as you write them.

*(Guidance note: the hypnotherapist should encourage discussion about each word/feeling as the client says the word)*

DOI: 10.4324/9781003468325-63

Sometimes it can be hard to find the right word to express a feeling. Some people find it easier to draw something – a shape – a colour – or a picture. Why not have a go at drawing now – a shape – a colour – or a picture. Use the arrow icon on the far right hand side of the toolbar and go to a fresh page. Then think again about how your regrets make you feel. I wonder what image comes into your head. Draw whatever image or images come into your head. Describe to me what you are drawing.

*(Guidance note: the hypnotherapist should encourage discussion about each image/drawing the client describes)*

Bring your attention back to the pencil icon. On the right hand side of the pencil icon you will see another icon – it is a rubber. It can rub things out – make them disappear completely. You might find that useful in a short while.

Next to the rubber icon – on the right hand side – you will see a camera icon. If you click on that it will open up the webcam. Do that now. See yourself on the screen. Tell me what you see.

*(Guidance note: if the client is reluctant to describe what they see, the hypnotherapist can use some of the prompts below)*

What do you see on the screen?
How does your face look?
What do you see in your face?
Is your face happy or sad?
What else do you see?

OK – click on the camera icon again and close the webcam. Next to the camera icon you will see a big S icon which is for saving; and a big D icon for deleting.

Now I would like you to use the arrow on the far right hand side of the toolbar again. Go forward and find a new white page. Before you start to work on this page it might be a good idea to take a break for a while. It is important not to stare at a screen for too long. You need to give your eyes a rest – you need to stretch your legs because it is not good to stay sitting in the same position for a long time – not moving – not going anywhere. So just get up and walk about a while. Take a bit of a break. Take a break from thinking about regrets. It is not good to think about regrets for long periods of time. It can be exhausting. It is good to walk away from regrets. I shall be quiet for a short time whilst you take a break.

*(Guidance note: the hypnotherapist should remain quiet for at least two minutes)*

Are you ready to come back to the computer? Good. Let's continue. You have already gone forward. You have a fresh, clean page in front of you. It is now time to think about your future. Think about what you want to happen in the future – after you have left the regrets behind. Because you are going to leave the regrets behind, aren't you? Use the pencil again to write down what you want – what you want to happen – what you want to do. Before you do that I wonder if you might want to change to a different colour for your writing. If you do want to make that change, do it now. Focus on the future. Write down what you want – what you want to happen – what you want to do. Tell me about your future.

*(Guidance note: the hypnotherapist should encourage discussion about the future)*

Use the arrow to go forward again to another fresh page. Keep thinking about your future. I wonder what image or images come into your head. Draw whatever image or images come into your head. Describe to me what you are drawing.

*(Guidance note: as before the hypnotherapist should encourage discussion about each image/drawing the client describes)*

So you can see the picture very clearly. You know exactly what you want – what you want to happen – what you want to do. You also know that you can achieve anything you really want to do. It is time now to rub out the past – rub out the regrets. Use the arrow on the left hand side to go backwards. Go backwards – go back to the words you wrote about how the regrets have made you feel – find that page. Now click on the rubber icon and rub out all those words. See the words being rubbed out – one by one. How good does that feel? The regrets are disappearing. You are feeling different in some way as the words disappear. Tell me when they have all gone and the page is completely blank. Now use the D icon and delete that page completely. Good – that page has been deleted forever.

*(Guidance note: sometimes the client has written words on more than one page. If this is the case the process of rubbing out and deletion will have to be repeated for each page which has been created)*

You are now left looking at the page with the images/drawings (*as appropriate*) you drew in relation to the regrets. It is time to rub them out. So click on the rubber icon again and rub out all those images/drawings. See the images/drawings being rubbed out – one by one. How good does that feel? The regrets are disappearing. You are feeling different in some way as the images/drawings disappear. Tell me when they have all gone and the page is completely blank. Now use the D icon again and delete that page completely. Good – that page has been deleted forever. There is nothing left to see from the past.

*(Guidance note: as above, sometimes the client has used more than one page to create images/drawings. If this is the case, the process of rubbing out and deletion will have to be repeated for each page which has been created)*

Now it is time to go forward. Look at the pages with the words and images/drawings you created about your future. You know what you want – what you want to happen – what you want to do – what changes you want to make. You can express what you want – what you want to happen – what you want to do – what changes you want to make. You can write about what you want – what you want to happen – what you want to do – what changes you want to make. You can draw what you want – what you want to happen – what you want to do – what changes you want to make. Look at those pages now. Look at them very carefully and see if you need to make any changes – add anything else. Take your time. Your future is important. Think about what you want – what you want to happen – what you want to do – what changes you want to make. Make any changes – make any additions – make your future just right. Tell me what you are doing.

Now you have the words to talk about your future. Now you can see your future. You will no longer feel regretful. The regrets have gone forever. They will no longer affect your life. You have the future to look forward to. So now it is time to save all those changes you have made and keep those pages safe, so you can come back and look at them any time you want to do so. So use the S icon and save those changes now and feel the change deep within you.

Let's see how you are looking now after making all those changes. Click on the camera icon and open the webcam. What do you see?

*(Guidance note: the hypnotherapist can use some of the following prompts if required)*

How do you look?
What has changed?
What is different?
How does your face look now?
What do you see in your face?
What else do you see?

*(Guidance note: the hypnotherapist should finish the session with some ego boosting)*

# Chapter 56

# High wire act

## Introduction

This script has been written for adults who may have regrets in regard to their job/career but more specifically about:

- Not having trained/studied previously and consequently lack confidence in themselves
- Not having applied for certain jobs – maybe because they think they are not good enough
- Not being ambitious in the past or currently
- Performance anxiety.

The script can also be used for children who lack confidence in themselves and may be struggling at school to learn/study or for children who have a fear of performing because they have made mistakes or forgotten something in the past. The purpose of the script is to build on confidence and embed the idea of performing well – being skilled – having no fear – being able to entertain – putting trust in other people – and working as a team.

## The script

I know you have had regrets about (*insert as appropriate*). I want to congratulate you on the fact that you have been working really hard on your regrets and making excellent progress. I think the time is right now to think about what you want to achieve for the future – how you want to perform. The regrets have been holding you back in many ways – stopping you from moving forward. So let's change that now so you move forwards and upwards.

I want you to imagine that you are part of a circus. This circus travels around the country and goes to many exciting places. Some towns and cities are familiar to the people working in the circus – other towns and cities are very new. You are now part of this circus. You perform on the high wire. Now all good acts practise a lot

DOI: 10.4324/9781003468325-64

before they perform, so I want you to go into the Big Top where the acts perform and stand in the circus ring.

You are standing right in the middle of the circus ring. Slowly turn around and look at all the empty seats. Now look up right above your head and you see a wire crossing overhead. You can see the ends of the wire are tied securely to poles which surround the platforms – the platforms where performers stand and wait. You are going to perform. You are going to perform on the high wire. You are an acrobat. Acrobats can do many spectacular things. They perform – they entertain – they can balance – they are agile – they can juggle – they can walk – skip – jump – cycle on a high wire. They can swing through the air from one platform to the other platform. You are able to do all of these things as an acrobat. You are confident. You are fearless. So show me what you can do.

Walk towards the rope ladder which is hanging down from one of the platforms. Start climbing the rope ladder – slowly and steadily. Breathe slowly in and out with each step you take upwards. As you continue to climb be aware of how good it feels to climb – to climb the rope ladder to the very top – climbing to the top without any hesitation at all – to experience exciting things when you get to the top. You find it so easy to climb to the top. You know what to do – you set your sights on the very top – and then start climbing. You are confident – skilled – you have no fear. You know you can climb to the top – when you are determined anything is possible.

You are going to perform and you will perform well. Keep climbing the rope ladder – slowly and steadily – breathing slowly in and out with each step upwards. You are nearly at the top now. Take a really deep breath before you step onto the platform. Step onto the platform now. Take another deep breath. It is important to keep your breathing nice and slow – filling your lungs with air – so you can perform and entertain.

Look around you from the platform. Look down into the circus ring and around it – look down and see the empty seats. Now look straight across from you and see the other platform. Look at the high wire that runs from the platform you are standing on to the platform on the other side. You are very high up – it feels exciting to be so high up. Notice at the side of the platform there is a swing – there are also some long poles. You are confident that you are going to perform well. You know you can perform well. You know you will do a good job and entertain many people in the future. The audiences will appreciate your performances.

Become conscious of your breathing again. You know it helps to focus on your breathing in order to prepare mentally for any performance. Take some deep breaths – nice and slow – feel the air going into your nostrils – and then down – deep into your lungs. You see some tennis balls have been left on the platform. You pick them up and start juggling. You are getting warmed up. You are good at juggling – juggling the balls – you are good at juggling lots of things in your life. You keep your eyes on the balls – throwing them up in the air and catching them. You juggle rhythmically and skilfully.

You are warmed up and ready to walk across the high wire. Take one of the shorter poles from the side of the platform. Get your balance. Concentrate. Now walk – off you go – walking steadily – confidently – perfectly balanced across the high wire. Keep going – head held up high – look straight across – keep going. Walking steadily – confidently – perfectly balanced. You are halfway there now. Keep going. Walking steadily – confidently – perfectly balanced. You have nearly reached the other platform – nearly there – now step onto the platform and put down the pole. Well done – a perfect performance.

You will see on the platform where you are now standing there is a swing and a selection of poles. Now choose a longer pole and walk back across the high wire. Get your balance. Concentrate. Now walk – off you go – walking steadily – confidently – perfectly balanced across the wire. Keep going – head held up high – look straight across – keep going. Walking steadily – confidently – perfectly balanced. You are halfway there now. Keep going. Walking steadily – confidently – perfectly balanced. You have nearly reached the other platform – nearly there – now step onto the platform and put down the pole. Well done – another perfect performance.

There are many different ways to cross the high wire. You have many different ways of performing and entertaining. So now you see a bicycle hanging on the side of the platform. Bring the bicycle onto the platform and get on it. Now you are going to cycle across the high wire. You can go at different speeds – fast – slow – whatever you want to do. All you have to do is keep your balance. If you have a little wobble you will stay calm – concentrate – get balanced again – and continue.

Ready – get your balance. Concentrate. Now cycle – off you go – cycling steadily – confidently – perfectly balanced across the high wire. Keep going – head held up high – look straight across – keep going. Cycling steadily – confidently – perfectly balanced. You are halfway there now. Keep going. Cycling steadily – confidently – perfectly balanced. You have nearly reached the other platform – nearly there – now cycle onto the platform. Well done – a perfect performance. In a moment you are going to cycle back across the high wire. You can go at different speeds – fast – slow – whatever you want to do. All you have to do is keep your balance. If you have a little wobble you will stay calm – concentrate – get balanced again – and continue.

Get your balance. Concentrate. Now cycle – off you go – cycling steadily – confidently – perfectly balanced across the high wire. Keep going – head held up high – look straight across – keep going. Cycling steadily – confidently – perfectly balanced. You are halfway there now. Keep going. Cycling steadily – confidently – perfectly balanced. You have nearly reached the other platform – nearly there – now cycle onto the platform. Well done – another perfect performance.

It is important to keep an audience entertained so you need to be able to perform a variety of skills. There will be times when you are performing when you might need to put your trust in other people. Several of you might be performing on the high wire at the same time – juggling – walking – jumping – skipping – cycling. You have to trust each other and work as a team.

Imagine performing using the swing. Imagine what it is like when it is just you using the swing to swing across from one platform to the other platform. Do that now – stand on the platform – grab hold of the bar on the swing – now step off the platform – swing back and forth – back and forth. You develop a steady swing – back and forth – back and forth. As you are swinging you see another person standing on one of the platforms. They are going to catch onto to your feet the next time you swing towards them and jump off the platform. Now they are hanging onto your feet and you are both swinging back and forth – back and forth. You have trust in each other. You work as a team. You keep swinging – performing – entertaining. Throughout the performance you keep your balance.

Now it is time to perform and entertain in front of an audience. Look down into the circus ring. See how the seats are filling up. You feel confident that you are going to perform well and entertain everyone in the audience. So what are you going to do?

*(Guidance note: the hypnotherapist can either repeat the performance above with the audience present OR if the client has spoken about their performance in a certain situation then further work can be undertaken in the session to rehearse their performance in a particular situation)*

# Index